T0136155

Globalizing AIDS

THEORY OUT OF BOUNDS

Edited by
Sandra Buckley
Michael Hardt
Brian Massumi

Globalizing AIDS

Cindy Patton

THEORY OUT OF BOUNDS, VOLUME 22

University of Minnesota Press
Minneapolis • London

An earlier version of chapter 3 appeared as "Performativity and Spatial Distinction: AIDS Education and the End of AIDS Epidemiology," in *Performativity and Performance*, ed. Eve Sedgwick and Andrew Parker (New York: Routledge, 1995); reprinted with permission from Routledge Press and the English Institute.

Published by the University of Minnesota Press
111 Third Avenue South, Suite 290
Minneapolis, MN 55401-2520
http://www.upress.umn.edu

Library of Congress Cataloging-in-Publication Data

Patton, Cindy, 1956–
    Globalizing AIDS / Cindy Patton.
        p.   ; cm. — (Theory out of bounds ; v. 22)
    Includes bibliographical references and index.
    ISBN 0-8166-3279-0 (HC : alk. paper) — ISBN 0-8166-3280-4 (PB : alk. paper)
    1. AIDS (Disease)—Social aspects.   2. AIDS (Disease)—Epidemiology.
3. World health.
    [DNLM: 1. Acquired Immunodeficiency Syndrome—epidemiology.
2. Politics.   3. World Health.   WC 503.41 P322g 2002]   I. Title.
II. Series.
RA643.8 .P38   2002
362.1'969792—dc21   2001008511

Printed in the United States of America on acid-free paper

The University of Minnesota is an equal-opportunity educator and employer.

12 11 10 09 08 07 06 05 04 03 02   10 9 8 7 6 5 4 3 2 1

Contents

Acknowledgments

Many people have had a hand in the making of this small book. Michael Warner, Katie Kent, Jennifer Stocking, Rhea Combs, Michael Shapiro, Andrew Parker, and Kathy Delfosse dealt directly with research, content, or copy, and I thank them especially for their patience with my notoriously bad spelling, neologisms, and quirky grammar. William Murphy and Richard Morrison of the University of Minnesota Press have been especially willing to go out on the syntactic limb to help retain the stylistic elements that, although perhaps nonstandard, have been important to me in trying to convey a sense of what it has been like to think at the margins of the moral and scientific crisis called AIDS. I also want to thank Mary Petty, whose insights gleaned from applying postmodern theory to clinical practice have deepened my understanding of the changing human experience of the epidemic. Her contribution has been practical (putting up with my moods during the long course of completing this project) and analytical (sharing her reflections of her own experience of caring for the dying while militating for the living). I also thank our dog Alex, who, although she may not differentiate among the various activities that involve typing, knows when to make me call it a day and go outside to play.

Emory University has been generous in offering me time and money to complete this project. In particular, I thank those responsible for the junior faculty award program and the Winship Distinguished Researchers program. I thank Tracy Allen-Blandon, who provided administrative support for me during a difficult year in our institute, which coincided with my last efforts to finish this book. She always had my back. I also thank Chen Kuan-Hsing and Ding Nai Fei, who made possible several extended trips to Taiwan to research HIV there and to present and receive feedback on the work here. I am sure that I have failed to thank important contributors to my life during the completion of this project. To you I apologize for omitting your names and I thank you.

Introduction

In the late 1960s, Canadian media theorist Marshall McLuhan popularized the phrase "global village," which captured the growing perception that for many people, mass media and transportation technologies had effectively reduced the size of the globe, irrevocably altering their sense of where they lived. Asserted at the height of the Vietnam War, the idea that the wonders of technology could transform the planet into a cozy village offered a less paranoid vision of Americans' place on spaceship earth than the images of secret invasion that had characterized Cold War ideology. Although the image of the global village ignored the political and economic differences among nations and cultures, it nevertheless suggested that the world's most powerful countries had a brotherly obligation to people who were, after all, really not all that different. This idea of harmony worked because the global village existed primarily as an imaginary hyperspace. Despite the myriad ways in which global travel concretely altered labor, tourism, defense, and domestic practices, it was the global news, entertainment, and information media, eventually including the Internet, that were crucial for conveying *ideas* about social and cultural similarity and difference. In the imagined space of the global village, we Baby Boomers were next to, but not actually touching, the many peoples and places we had, during our paranoid Cold War childhood, discovered in our *Weekly Reader.*

Imagine our surprise when our Age of Aquarius ended with a frightening new disease. The hyperspace of the

global village confronted the profound materiality of ailing bodies slowly sharing—*communicating*—a new, fatal
illness. In the face of a threat that could not be confined
to any single place, the dark side of global brotherhood
reemerged. Global proximity no longer promised won-
drous cultural explorations; rather, it seemed to facilitate
the spread of exotic new diseases that were not only deadly
to individual bodies but also threatening to the body politic:
to its humanitarian ideals, its emerging global economy,
and even, according to right-wing pundits, its ability to
reproduce biologically. The practical realities of bodily
contact, realities that had evaporated in the mediated embrace of global brotherhood, now seemed closer than close,
realer than real—corpo-real. There were three levels of response to the challenge the tiny virus posed to our sense
of place and our sense of safety: national, international or
supranational, and local.

1. *National.* By the mid-1980s, more than fifty countries had created new border-control regulations or had
invoked existing ones in an effort to get rid of or prevent
the entry of potentially infected persons. HIV Ab testing,
newly available in 1985, only provided a scientific veneer
to policies based on national, religious, racial, gender, or
class stereotypes.[1] Interest in cultural difference was transformed into suspicion that people who were in any way
different harbored dangerous and contagious diseases. In
the global village of frantic neighbors, national borders
took on a new role as they falsely promised of safety from
disease.

2. *International or supranational.* Organizations, such
as the United Nations or the World Health Organization

(WHO), and international news-gathering agencies stepped in to describe the big picture. Global policy groups sought widely applicable solutions to a disease phenomenon that seemed, incredibly enough, to have appeared almost simultaneously in disparate cultures and apparently unconnected places around the globe. Despite the fact that all signs pointed to a handful of major cities in the United States as the source of the disease, international media cloaked itself in scientific language and endlessly quoted the premature remarks of AIDS science luminaries, like Luc Montagne, who asserted that AIDS must have started in Africa.

By the late 1980s, the WHO employed equally obfuscatory ideas about risk behaviors to produce an epidemiological mapping of the world that continues to profoundly affect how we understand AIDS as a *pandemic*. The pattern of AIDS incidence associated with North America and Europe, where identified cases were originally predominantly found among homosexually active men and injecting drug users of both sexes, was called Pattern One. That of Africa, where cases were initially identified among heterosexually active but non-drug-injecting people, was called Pattern Two. Pattern Three was defined not by the demographics of its cases but by their location in a space-time framework: where "AIDS arrived late," that is, principally Asia.

Although the simple scheme of three world patterns may originally have had broad scientific and heuristic value in preparing for a pandemic, it quickly took on a narrative life of its own, offering supranational policy makers and news reporters a veneer of scientific objectivity for what were essentially racist and class-disadvantaging represen-

tations of local epidemics. Almost immediately, the pseu-
doscientific label "African AIDS" circulated with more
resonance, and perhaps more credibility, than did the official WHO term, "Pattern Two," to describe the spread
of the disease in places where cases related to heterosexual intercourse seemed to predominate. This recycling of
very old racist ideas that alleged unchecked sexuality in
Africa, or among black people generally, was devastating
for local activism in both Africa and North America. In
many African nations, the Global Programme on AIDS
(GPA), national health ministries, nongovernmental organizations (NGOs), and local activists promoted a "return
to monogamy" instead of exploring the complex class, migration, and cultural patterns that concretely framed the
epidemic.

In developing countries, colonialism and modernization were commonly blamed for local epidemics. But although the social and economic relations that undergird
the epidemic did in general develop alongside colonial
and postcolonial or modern political regimes, from the
standpoint of local action, broad political critiques are in-
sufficient bases on which to develop a public health response. The heated battle between those who cloak racism
in scientific language and those who attack the colonialist
legacy still present within science and global health management quickly resulted in a political and scientific gap
between the two sides; both lacked a detailed analysis of
local health delivery practices and ignored the political
and sociosexual economy of decolonizing or democratiz-
ing places. This fatal misdirection of science and politics

did not affect just the people of Uganda, Kenya, and Cameroon, the major African locales and nation-states involved in these early debates. In the United States, when the media finally, in about 1987, saw fit to report the high number of AIDS cases among African Americans and black immigrants in Europe and North America, the affected individuals were assumed to be heterosexual: sexually deviant in the *form* of their relations rather than in their sex-gender objects. The demographics of AIDS did not prompt a sharp analysis of the systemic and localized racism and poverty in some of the world's wealthiest nations; rather, in the case of the U.S. media, the image of an African continent of seething sex and rampant death was simply relocated to describe America's black communities, now said to be "like" villages in Africa.

These problematic cultural imaginings corresponded neatly to the incidence maps generated by official health monitors. When the WHO created materials to help the media explain the epidemic, they simplified science and tried to unify the prevention message. In the mistaken conviction that folk terms would speed the uptake of facts, the media further dumbed down what was intended as lifesaving information. When scientific findings, already marred by incomplete understanding of the disease process and by inadequate frameworks for understanding the social lives of those studied—gay men, sex workers, colonial subjects, women—were passed through these circuits of reinterpretation, the result was widespread, unchecked, and socially powerful misinterpretation. A particularly devastating example is the way late 1980s scientific research on viral strain variation was represented and then popularly interpreted: Instead of explaining that there are hundreds of small genetic differences between isolates of HIV,[2] few if any of which correlate with symptomatic differences, the media suggested that an early-identified but not well-understood cluster of West African cases "proved" that AIDS had started "in Africa." The macrolevel idea of patterns of transmission now combined with virologists' efforts at characterizing the retrovirus and produced a deeply problematic popular belief that science had proven that different modes of transmission were linked with viral strains of greater and lesser potency. The continuing reinforcement of the idea that African cases were different—first sociosexually and later virally—influenced mainstream North Americans' conviction that it was virtually impossible for "ordinary people" (now encompassing straight, native-born, white, and probably middle-class folks) to contract HIV during "ordinary intercourse." This latter activity probably meant "missionary-position sex," but it was rarely clear what activities were proper to the "ordinary" person and whether, for example, individuals who engaged in "nonordinary" sex were thereby somehow liable to transmit HIV even when they engaged in "ordinary intercourse." Just as there was confusion over whether male-male intercourse was a risk practice or the defining activity of a risk group, there was confusion over who needed to consider safe sex, and those who were encouraged to see themselves as "ordinary" or as members of the "heterosexual community" were discouraged from thinking much about it.

This confused conjoining of an erroneous understanding of the HIV cluster in West Africa and the mis-association of Africanness and sexual extraordinariness played out in an especially ugly way in Canada in 1993. In a case that received wide and sensational reportage (including the 1995 *Trial without End: A Shocking Story of Women and AIDS* by Canadian liberal feminist June Callwood), an "African" man was accused of recklessly infecting others. The reportage on the cluster of "heterosexual infections" attributed to Mr. Charles Ssenyonga in the criminal trial did not emphasize the importance of safe sex among heterosexuals; instead, it pointed to his race and national origin as the "risk" factors. Combining both the sociosexual and viral difference theories, the media suggested that it was not heterosexual intercourse but Mr. Ssenyonga's "super viral load" and exceptional sexual abilities that had caused HIV transmission. This kind of reportage suggested that for the white, middle-American or middle Canadian, cases among Africans and African Canadians or African Americans are as remote and unpreventable as the represented epidemic in "Africa." This increasingly exaggerated image of African and African American difference rendered America's black ghetto, although in reality proximate, phantasmically distant: Linking the WHO's global nomenclature with local situations and policies—sometimes even in the work of activists—led to the widely publicized conviction that black inner city youths were "unreachable."

3. *Local.* The third reaction to HIV occurred in many individual locales. "Local response" conjures images of earnest people living with AIDS (PLWA)[3] organizations;

corporatized, even bureaucratic, AIDS service organizations (ASOs); and confrontational groups like ACT UP—all fighting in their own way against government and scientific inaction and indifference. But although this image of Big Science being begged, co-opted, or harassed has its roots in real experience with the governance of medical knowledge production and care distribution, it naively suggests that if local doctors and policy makers can just be made to listen to people living with HIV, they will develop compassion and join activists in exerting pressure on governments and policy makers "higher up" at the national and international levels. But as I will argue here, merely incorporating the "voice of the people" does not change the relationship between medical science and the bodies it describes. Long-term AIDS activists are, of course, acutely aware that the politics of health—especially the complex construction and distribution of scientific knowledge—are misunderstood by the false-consciousness-grassroots-up theory of change. The march-on-science model rests on the false assumption that scientific and popular knowledges of the body are separate. Instead, AIDS activist groups like ACT UP (AIDS Coalition to Unleash Power) carried an academic dispute about the social construction of science into the streets, inviting other groups of "sufferers" to reconstruct their recognized or unrecognized experience in and against biomedical terms, a process of knowledge hybridization that is in its turn now studied by academics.[4] For individual participants in both local and global political processes, AIDS activism has been an important and world-changing experience of questioning and reshaping how body-knowledge is given to, reinterpreted within, and applied to real disease processes. Through the efforts of uniquely situated PLWAs from the United States, the top policy makers at the WHO did indeed have the opportunity to meet with a wide range of people immediately and directly affected by HIV. In the late 1980s, activists from many countries helped persuade the WHO's GPA to speak out against antigay and antiprostitute discrimination, to advise against the use of HIV antibody testing as a form of immigration screening, and to support expanded definitions of AIDS. Tragically, the United States did not honor the efforts of its own citizens, men and women who worsened their physical condition through long hours of research, presentations, and hectic travel schedules. Instead, the United States refused to adopt most of the policies proposed by the GPA, which the U.S. government had financially supported and endorsed.

The story of early AIDS activism shows in relief the extraordinarily complex interplay between different kinds of local and nationwide campaigning, on the one hand, and the responses of official government and medical bodies, on the other. But as I will continually stress here, the first "activism" was conducted not by ACT UP and not even by self-identifying people living with HIV. The first resistance occurred before AIDS was even given a name. Everywhere that someone was sick, individuals and networks banded together for mutual aid. Without having a diagnostic label, without even recognizing that their complex of symptoms would remain a mystery to their doctors, the first people sick with what would soon be named AIDS entered the many different kinds of medical systems around the world and quickly learned and shared important information about their bodies' experiences. In most cases, these individuals were not the patients for whom the care delivery systems were designed, and not just because they were presenting the leading edge of a new, even perhaps a new *kind of,* epidemic. Whether they were sex workers in Kinshasa, African immigrants in Brussels, or gay men in Los Angeles, these early affected persons had already been marked as different and were deemed troublesome by the medical systems they attended. Paradoxically, as people matching existing stereotypes appeared within the administrative systems that use medical care for policing, the collision between individual physical need and social desire to control allowed those original cases to become visible to the world medical community. Because surveillance systems were already on the alert for sexual "deviants" and unwanted immigrants, officials noticed and quickly told their colleagues of their mysteriously ill or inexplicably dead patients. Inaccurate as these initial, discriminatory understandings were, they formed the prerequisite of modern epidemiology: They connected illness with a population whose shared location, traits, or practices promised to yield clues to the origin and dynamics of a disease.

The particular images and concepts of AIDS that emerged from this early thinking framed and structured the issues addressed by the several styles of activism that quickly emerged: issues of antidiscrimination law, patient access and care, innovations in scientific thinking and processes, and health-system reform. However, although the problems faced by PLWAs were in many ways universal, and although global activism was strongly influenced by that in the United States, it nevertheless operated in different geopolitical corridors and had different local meanings and effects. Efforts to improve access and fight discrimination were often local, aimed at the *specific* cluster of prejudices held by the systems and people who managed HIV in a particular *place*. On the other hand, GPA efforts to stimulate both government and nongovernment responses to the epidemic caused new NGOs to form and meet with representatives of such traditional aid groups as the Red Cross in order to formulate proposals for worldwide antidiscrimination laws and to share local and constituency-based models for coping with HIV and the attendant social problems. U.S.-based AIDS activism initially emerged in response to the particular problems of U.S.-style, market-based medicine and to the debates about sexuality and race within Reaganite America, and in the context of a Rainbow Coalition politics that was in shambles. But this response became a model for other people in other places—even when their historical situation was radically different. For example, relatively financially stable emerging democracies, like Taiwan, already had universal medical care for PLWAs. In Taiwan, the question was less access to care than the consequences—as a kind of "coming out"—of accessing that care.

Experience, Knowledge

Despite revisions in global thinking about AIDS—much of that change forced by activists—the contours of media representation, policy, research, and activism are, I argue, still formed from and publicized through the shifting positions of local, national, and global organizations. Ideas flow from localities to national and supranational organizations and back, through both regular and intermittent routes, such as the media, the World Wide Web, international conferences, and random visitors. The raggedness of these various kinds of global information flow is not just a policy issue—not just a question of how to manage the globalization of media and information. It is, in addition, the very fabric of our understanding of the epidemic and of our place in it. It is not that the local is real and the rest is abstract: We *experience* the national and the international dimensions of our world. In fact, non-face-to-face spaces are extremely important elements of reality, for activists, for researchers, and for people living with HIV. To acknowledge only local knowledge suggests that we cannot understand any situation we have not directly experienced and ignores the role of other registers of experience in helping us conceptualize, interpret, and realize our particular situation. People living with HIV have struggled with how to form coalitions across vast differences in culture, economic status, gender, ethnic and national affiliation, and sensibilities toward medical systems. Their locally specific and universal experiences have been globally publicized, influencing all levels of policy and the most personal understandings of an individual life with AIDS. If one does not have HIV, the people one knows and the stories one reads offer insight into the issues faced by those who are labeled "HIV+" and must routinely submit to the medical and social system. But similarly, if one has HIV, one's sense of place and time are profoundly influenced by the stories of earlier PLWAs and PLWAs elsewhere. Very few Westerners of either serostatus have gone to a mining town in Zaire to discover personally what having HIV means there. And yet most of us have voiced strong critiques of our country's policies toward developing countries' health care systems. Researchers and clinicians from developing countries have offered their experiences to people from economically more powerful countries hoping to make clearer the dynamics of health care delivery in economically and politically disempowered places. Even without holding exactly the same form of knowledge about other places as we hold about our own, we can and do have a sense of *pandemic*.

I describe spaces of knowledge primarily as different ways of, to somewhat expand Benedict Anderson's term, *imagining community*: from face-to-face contact to mediated hyperspace and everything in between. The differences that flow from competing and commingling knowledge/community situations, much in the critical eye of those concerned with globalization, are only one axis of concern in this volume. The second, perhaps less assessed differences among varied knowledge/community situations concern the discursive and practical interrelation of science and people. Here, too, what is real, what is understood as knowledge, is not separable into what we sense directly and scientific knowledge. At the beginning of what we now cast as the space-time of pandemic, individuals lived the problems in their bodies and with the medical system without benefit of any unifying terms, either the diagnosis—AIDS—or its ancillary, empowering, translocal expression of experience, "people living with AIDS." Something very significant happened in the apparently simple act of assigning a name to a disease process, and then again in the process of building collective action from the personal experiences of illness grouped under that name. The acceptance of HIV symptoms as a disease syndrome and the willingness to search for and find a cause reflect the insistence by the first people to fall ill that something *outside* their bodies was causing the changes within. Now that we see the extent of the epidemic, it seems inevitable that science would take an interest. But malign neglect has been the norm in a century of miracle cures. Millions of people have suffered or died of starvation and preventable diseases. Especially when we are talking about stigmatized people, we should never consider science's interest a foregone conclusion. Science, however moral, brilliant, and humanitarian its practitioners, is necessarily imbricated in politics. I will largely leave it to others to detail the political economy of scientific research, taking up instead the sociopolitical nature of scientific thought as it is popularly narrated. A brief example should clarify the line of inquiry I will follow here, an inquiry that accuses neither scientists of becoming improperly politicized nor politicians of callously appropriating science. Instead, I conceive of science and politics as expressions of meandering styles of conceiving a world.

Two politically opposite quasi-scientific interests made recognition of the early AIDS cases possible. In the United States, the first recognized cases were among gay men who had access to health care. Their doctors were perplexed at the men's illnesses or deaths and had adopted a new, antipathologizing understanding of sexuality, at least enough to refrain from assuming that homosexual men were simply biologically unviable. This change in attitude hinted at the extent to which political mobilization of stigmatized groups affected medical thought, and it foreshadowed the definitive role that explicitly politicoscientific responses would play in the epidemic. But soon, other cases—among immigrants, users of illegal drugs, and poor people who were already under scrutiny by health-policing systems— were recognized as having the same illness. Here, it was suspicion of difference rather than mobilization by the oppressed that enabled the preoccupation with illness that resulted in the recognition of this second class of cases. By 1983, both of these reasons for noticing—new, politically positive visibility and inability to hide from health authorities—were inextricably meshed in the surveillance and education practices that accompanied the epidemic.

However convinced the early people with AIDS and their doctors were that something was wrong, only when epidemiology could frame a category was it possible to officially attach a set of researchable symptoms to a scientifically derived name. Assigning a name was crucial to the political response: The methodical nature of Western medicine and the degree to which modern society is medicalized means that without the procedures and sanctions of official medicine, expressions of bodily experiences and complaints are not considered real, sometimes not even by the sufferer. In order for science, policy, representation, criticism, and activism to have a space of engagement, there had to be a name that could roughly incorporate—albeit through a changing definition—the widely dispersed, culturally distinct, and symptomatically varied bodies. At least as it stands now, we can struggle over our involvement in the medical process, but we must submit our bodies to medical science if we are to have any hope of access to the potentially lifesaving resources that modern science may produce. Without a common language, medical researchers cannot work with us and we cannot activate the specialized knowledge that might help us repair the damage done by a virus. The strange paradox of AIDS activism has been that it emerged from a sense of not being heard, but it is partly voiced in the scientific language and ways of thinking that have now merged, almost imperceptibly, with local languages and community ways of thinking.

For two decades, medical people, people living with HIV, people concerned about the organization of health care, people struggling for the rights and dignity of stigmatized people, and people who are all of these at once have worked to alleviate the suffering and improve the lives of people who have contracted a newly discovered virus and to help those who are as yet uninfected remain so. Many people are worn out or cynical or even ready to abandon the general commitment to the goal of well-executed science quickly delivering its product to individuals who are treated with dignity in communities that are recognized as unique cultures. Some people are even ready to abandon the effort to provide locally meaningful education to stem the tide of new cases among the young people who are the emerging pool of new homes for a deadly virus.

But instead of abandoning hope, we must continually reevaluate the concepts through which we understand HIV, looking closely at how the multiple levels of experience and the multiple forms of knowledge interrelate and change over time. The epidemic moves and changes, leveling off for a period in one group in one place, say, among Baby

Boomer gay men in San Francisco, while intensifying in another group in another place, say, among young Latin women in Los Angeles or young gay men in Paris, or appearing in new places, such as parts of Asia and the Pacific Islands or small towns in the U.S. Midwest. Each of these groups lives in a complex world of media, national policy, international organizations, and local physicians and researchers. How each group experiences and comes to understand HIV will be different from the way the others do and different again from the way it was understood by even culturally similar people who were infected in earlier periods of the epidemic. How a seronegative male drug injector or gay man in a hard-hit area experiences the fact that he is not infected is very different from the understanding of uninfected people who have never imagined themselves to be at risk because they see themselves as leading "ordinary lives." Each of these understandings is different again from those of a gay man or sex worker or "ordinary person" who, at the late date of 2000, is among the first to discover he or she is infected in his or her own small corner of the world, whether that is in the Solomon Islands or in Tiny Town, Queensland, or in a suburb of London.

The melding of local knowledge and global perspectives and of personal experience and scientific research that got us to the present is both useful and problematic. Our task now is to reconsider what it means to think in terms of community, nation, and globe and to understand who can be empowered by such concepts and who will be excluded. How do different ways of locating ourselves enable mutual understanding, and how do they stand in the way of coalition building? Perhaps even more challenging, how do we recognize as individual, while still coordinating and organizing, the experiences of people affected by the epidemic in different ways—not only as seropositive versus seronegative or in low-incidence versus high-incidence places, but also as frontline workers, scientists, and educators and as people with differing ties to family, friends, profession, culture, and nation?

One thing this pandemic reveals is that everyone on this planet is interconnected—not always in ways that are clear or direct, but in ways that have medical and political consequences that inexorably unfold. Our situation is far more complex than even a perverse reading of McLuhan's prescient words suggests. It is vital to disentangle some of the strands of medical and spatial thinking that form the grid through which interconnected global actors understand the situation faced *here, now*. This volume spins on two axes: first, the relationship between global and local, and second, the relationship between two ways of narrating the science of AIDS. Various authors have examined the mechanisms through which AIDS became an actual pandemic and a metaphor for globalization processes. Others have examined the crisis in scientific thinking that HIV and its eradication have produced. By looking simultaneously at medical thoughtstyles and the trajectories of activism and policy through local and global communities, I hope to shed light on why a "global solution" may be impossible and why the legacies of colonialism and modernization allow for the spectacular and insidious recycling of racist, sexist, xenophobic, and homophobic ideas as though they were "scientific." In the course of the first chapters, I will distinguish between two models of thought about disease and its movement. Though overlapping in concepts and in institutional development, these models nevertheless propose rather different explanations for the cause, mobility, and eradication of disease. Furthermore, I hope to break down several cases in which contradictory explanations came to seem reasonable and which, internationalized through governmental and scientific institutions, became the commonplace knowledge that we experience as "global AIDS." The route to untangling this connotative sense of "AIDS" will take us into some rather abstract discussions of language and of geography. However, if activism is to retain its critical edge, its various capacities to touch individual lives and influence global policy, it is important, at this juncture, to reexamine how the medical models of thought have been both challenged and reemployed to pull activism in one direction or to deflect it into another. Activist projects must be developed and criticized not just for their cultural sensitivity, for their local productiveness, for their fit with postcolonial health managers' ideas about the state of nations' development, or even for their visibility in the grid of the UN AIDS programs. We must also place the concerns, successes, and failings of activism in relation to the struggle over medical thought.

CHAPTER 1

Critical Bodies

From the epidemic's dawn, AIDS activists have been deeply aware of the ways in which the body is constituted through biomedicine and social science and painfully cognizant of how that body is policed through the public policies and health-education programs developed from these research disciplines. Nevertheless, bodies—we—are also desperately dependent on precisely these scientific institutions and practices for any hope of medical care, antidiscrimination statutes, or prevention programs. Thus, activists and cultural critics concerned with the epidemic are in the precarious situation of challenging the way AIDS is described and then policed while simultaneously inhabiting bodies constituted through those descriptions. We live the material effects of the representations and policies into which we have sought to intervene. But although wrenching, this complicated, sometimes masochistic refusal to be compliant objects of scientific debate has enabled theoretical and practical responses that are exciting, volatile, and surprisingly effective.

From the first moment of recognition that there was a new epidemic, brave souls placed their bodies and their faces in front of the media, medical congresses, governmental investigative committees, and their friends and family to ask that their names be spoken, that the individual and collective experiences of those whom the disease claimed be recognized—*first*. Men and women around the world offered hope to others through these now-unfathomable acts of courage. Later, the spare, graphic eloquence of the 1986 "silence = death" poster articulated the wordless numbing terror felt by anonymous gay New Yorkers and soon became an emblem for another kind of activism that spread around the world.

Two waves of AIDS activism[1] rising from the gay communities in the West have claimed a range of victories: The first five years of the epidemic witnessed the establishment of community-based groups that secured ongoing visibility for the people most directly affected by the changing epidemic. By about 1987, anarchic protests known as "treatment activism" had forced a new understanding of people who had contracted HIV: They had become active participants—consumers of medical care—rather than passive victims. By hammering away at soft points in scientific nomenclature, drug marketing, and ethical frameworks, this form of activism helped prompt researchers and ethics boards in the United States to streamline drug trials. Experimental drugs were more quickly and more widely available for those who wished to try them. HIV/AIDS came to be understood as a chronic disease, a spectrum disease.[2] Individuals who were clearly sick, even disabled, but who had not fit the original, highly restrictive definition of AIDS could now receive the insurance and social service benefits denied them under the earlier definition. In the early 1990s, epidemiologists and clinicians finally agreed to broaden the official definition of AIDS to include gynecological symptoms and low T-cell counts, even in the absence of clinically definitive opportunistic infection.[3]

Doctors now believed what seropositive women knew: They were in fact sick. Their gynecological symptoms were taken seriously and were assessed and treated in the context of their immunodeficiency. When gynecological symptoms were placed on the continuum of disease progression, researchers could no longer exclude women from antiviral trials. They had to reconsider whether usually effective treatments could be modified to meet the demands of gynecological problems that were secondary to this form of immune suppression. From the standpoint of early diagnosis, clinicians were now more aware that gynecological abnormalities might indicate an underlying, otherwise unexpressed HIV infection. The changes that activism forced in names and categories—in the *discourse* through which scientists produced knowledge about the new disease—had direct, rapid, and material effects on the lives of those who already had "it."

The discursive changes wrought by activists also offered a critical perspective on the epidemic, even for those who fought back in more traditionally visible ways. Ironically, just when many liberal academics were complaining that Michel Foucault's descriptions of discourses and institutions could not produce real politics because they erased individual agency, AIDS activists forged such analyses into a new kind of politics that blasted institutions' extraordinary and anonymous power to name and categorize.

It is common now to imagine that AIDS activism began with the rise of ACT UP after 1987. But that history relies on an idea of activism that valorizes the most theatrically oppositional work: street theater, posters, demonstrations, disruptions. Despite their rather different styles of criticizing the government, both leftist academics and the media made a fetish of ACT UP, as if its impoliteness, its *obscenity*, cut through a web of slickly crafted lies to reveal something basic about the experience of illness in the face of indifference. Certainly, ACT UP reintroduced agitprop into a rather bland political scene in which Ronald Reagan's idiotic B-film acting counted as "great communication." But activism *began* when the first living person was acknowledged to have an unnamed but recognizable syndrome and had to cope with a hostile medical system. Before ACT UP could make minimal sense as a coalition raging against government and industry inaction, affected bodies had to accumulate into a class, and the disease that bound them together had to find a name.

I can only barely describe to those who were not yet involved what it was like in 1982: the near impossibility of getting the attention of the medical and policy empire, the closed-book existence of people living in the hazy shadow state we were encouraged to view as unerringly fatal and which we soon learned to call "AIDS." In the early 1980s, we compared the response to AIDS to the responses to the then most impressive, recently identified diseases: Legionnaires' disease and toxic shock syndrome. Such comparisons seem bizarre now, but they hint at what it was like to lodge the charge that society was unresponsive to a disease syndrome that was not yet acknowledged with a name. Now, we compare the invisibilities of that time to the current ones: We suggest that what women or people of color living with HIV experience today is like what the first people experienced. But however wretched their conditions, the disenfranchised of today can at least partially express their situation, even if they must insert their story into a history of the epidemic that recognizes them, but only by obliterating the deep trauma of their loss, a condition the late Jean-François Lyotard (1988) called *le différend*, the situation in which a person not only suffers a harm but is deprived of the means to express "it."[4] In fact, he suggested, the very presence of victims raises questions about the authenticity of their experiences: If their traumas were so great, then why are they left to tell about them? This gap, or residual wrong, this difference between what was done and what the reparations system can offer in return, is lodged as a deep ache that we all feel, victim or not: We can offer some forms of compensation, but we know no justice that can right the wrong of silenced trauma.

In practical terms, although the media now presume that someone is being ignored, they apply a standard, generic analysis of oppression to represent any pleas of the ignored. The specificity of suffering and even the possibilities for redress are written out of the picture as readers and audiences, encouraged to wallow in the feeling that someone has been left out, are distracted from facing their own implication in the complex morality of giving or not giving care, recompense, or even a fair hearing. I am not suggesting that the wrongs suffered by the first people with AIDS were worse than those suffered by people today. Remember, the first to die were men and women of many countries and colors who suffered many routes of infection: It is not *their* fault that science and the media mainly presented the most privileged among them, white gay sons of middle America. No story of AIDS has ever been adequate; no story of trauma can ever really tell the truth; all the individual accounts have been mobilized in aid of an international passion play in which the wronged can only pantomime their suffering to make it palatable to a world that cannot stand to face its actions. Thus, rather than *ranking* suffering—which is, at any rate, a narrative move within the AIDS story that I am here trying to critique—I want to consider the moral and politicoscientific cost of so quickly finding a place for the crimes against humanity that were committed before The Name.[5] Only when we stand and face the unnarratable horrors can we appreciate the modes of redress that have been left in abeyance because the story of AIDS we now tell leads us to misrecognize the utter contingency of the political responses we have known.

Some will say that I am simply asking to "tell a different story," as if that would make everyone see the truth because my "different story" is scientifically more accurate or politically more expedient. On the contrary: I do not believe that the politicoscientific representation masks a "real" experience. I will try to show in the section "Thinking without Proper Nouns" that, much as we use religious narrative to frame personal experience and social order, we today use and reshape science to make and break our corporeality. I differ, too, from those who believe that science is utterly fabricated. I want to take seriously the interrelation of collective mental constructions—what Ludwig Fleck called "thoughtstyles"—and a world of constraints and possibilities that we still have trouble thinking of as other than "natural."[6] In short, I am trying, along with other critics and analysts of the construction of scientific and popular knowledge, to edge my way out of a modernist way of thinking that erroneously splits the ideal and the material, that conceives of science as the incremental uncovering of a world about which we will ultimately have perfect knowledge. Of course, most scientists working in physics—the ur-science—believe that the world is a flux of accidents and possibilities and that the present is the result of only one trajectory among them. But the rest of us cling to the notion that there is something fixed, and that this "reality" lies outside of our social and political— including politicoscientific—processes. The early naming of AIDS will help clarify the position I take with respect to science. By raising questions about the political foreclosure—even despite scientific criticism of the category "AIDS"—that the event of naming effected, I hope to honor those who lost their lives before we had a way to place them in the Story of AIDS.

Thinking without Proper Nouns

A powerful history, organized around the theme of unresponsiveness, now seems to be the truth. The structural elements of the story are compelling, naturalized through the distorting then-now format of such popular accounts as the Home Box Office (HBO) production *And the Band Played On* or Jonathan Demme's *Philadelphia*, or in countless speeches by Liz Taylor, which appear in magazines ranging from *Time* to *People*. This is the history to which nearly everyone now assents, and it has been hard in the making. It is certainly a much more compassionate story than the "AIDS is God's will" genocidal story presented by some on the religious right. But it succeeds as *the* story because all involved can mark their exit from the march of excuses, official inaction, and petty prejudice and glory in their entry into AIDS awareness. In a bastardized version of Elisabeth Kubler-Ross's *On Death and Dying*, narrations of AIDS took labels for individuals' reactions to death and applied them as collective reactions to political conditions. Imagining infinite and telescoping cycles of ignorance, denial, and acceptance, we pause at way stations in a tragedy of moral regret instead of facing the harsher truth that systematic death is happening, *now*. The sentimentality a story of denial and acceptance affords suggests that if we can imagine the realities of AIDS now, we can transport ourselves into the past, into someone else's experience. Instead of demanding that we *do something*, we imagine ourselves in the place of victims, whom we presume we can save. We are really just sparing ourselves the truth: Our uniforms are marked by stripes, not by stars.

I invoke this past before The Name, this time that was obliterated when science pronounced that something called "AIDS" existed, because the particular ideas that are now an almost unshakable representational frame emerged before The Name. It is easy to imagine that "AIDS" came first, that it was a narrative beginning instead of an ideological end, the moment in which contradictory scientific and moral ideas became encapsulated in a single acronym. Perhaps a full-scale assault on science, an absolute rather than strategic refusal to be the passive bodies of epidemiology, might have produced a lifesaving moral crisis in Americans' relationship to their science, a crisis grave enough to have placed us in a truly brave new world. It is unclear to me now, still, how that would have improved the treatment of those first people or produced the cure that, I am afraid, will always be a fantasy. But I must honor that time when specific bodies, known as numbers to epidemiologists, by name to those of us acquainted with them, were wronged in a way that could not and still cannot be easily expressed. If we forget those bodies, we will never understand what we are hearing behind the poignant utterances of their successors today.

If I sound nostalgic—as I have sometimes been accused—it is because I can only stutter the unspeakable memory of a time with no history. The fragment I write here, anamnesis, is my only possible homage to a time, like the times of revolutionaries struggling under martial law or other more obvious forms of state oppression, in which the lessons of only a year or two are lost because the people who committed their bodies to those politics are dead. Even if I cannot describe the scope of what they felt and did, I can remind us to stop forgetting—for a moment. But I am not longing for a return to some idyllic time of pure politics that never was; rather, I hope to call forth a future, or rather, to stop us from foreclosing a next moment that only scientific positivism and blind politics believe can be known in advance. I am not being utopian—as I have also been accused—because I do not believe we can imagine our way to a brighter future. Instead, I suggest that we take seriously, that we *feel*, the utter contingency of this thing we now cannot but think of as "AIDS." It is, I think, impossible to write the history of the time before The Name, but we do not have to live with the present as if the path that led us here was not a contingent one, as full of accident as good intention.

Organizing before The Name was in many ways the most grotesquely essentialist form of organizing imaginable: a brilliant and painful example of what political commentators now call "strategic essentialism." In those days, attaining visibility was crucial. We were desperate to ensure that unrecognized people did not simply disappear, uncounted, dead from an unnamed medical syndrome with an unknown cause. We had to prove we existed in order to prove people were dying. We had to go to doctors and hospitals and government officials and say, in so many words, "We are gay people. We vote. You know we are your constituency"—the sort of political practice it is now almost clichéd to criticize. But even this bald essentialism by no means guaranteed success. Those men and women might just as easily have slipped away, remembered only by loved ones whose own survival might be compromised by the act of calling attention to the deaths. Who knew, in 1982, that an entire nation of queers would be willing to stand shoulder to shoulder so that the gaps that represented the dead could be visible against a sea of the living?

Under a Sign

We now know that gay communities' visibility in the 1980s was an effect of the economic and social infrastructures they had built up in the United States since World War II. After weathering the House Committee on Un-American Activities trials and government witch-hunts for homosexuals, by the mid-1960s, the gay liberation movement was ready to join the general movements toward freedom. Almost immediately, a right-wing backlash directly attacked lesbian and gay efforts to attain civil liberties, and the media diluted the movement's political power by presenting sexual liberation as the quintessential absurdity of the me generation. But lesbian and gay enclaves forged economic, social, and political ties as they increasingly occupied urban space. They became a business bloc, a consumer bloc, a voting bloc. By the early 1980s, when the epidemic first appeared, homotopias *looked* like communities. But since lesbian and gay rights were—still are—a dream, it was difficult to appeal for governmental response to the new epidemic on the basis of distributional justice. Instead, grassroots AIDS activism transformed existing organizations and friendship networks into autonomous and freestanding social service and medical units: the Gay Men's Health Crisis (GMHC) in New York, the AIDS Action Committee in Boston, STOP AIDS in Los Angeles, the San Francisco AIDS Foundation, and soon, the People with AIDS Coalition. These first groups arose explicitly because the government was doing little more than counting cases, but they also cemented and reproduced the bonds that corresponded to the form of community envisioned by minoritarian rhetoric. They were not *of* the state, but via the rhetoric and ideas of civil rights, they demanded recognition *by* the state. By the end of the 1980s, homotopias were no longer radical, and queers imagined themselves to be a Queer Nation.[7] If this deeply enabling notion of community was to survive, they could not very well retreat as the government begrudgingly responded. Instead, many of these groups combined government grants and corporate and community donations to became large, solidly financed, nonprofit organizations, much like the agencies that addressed other health or social-welfare issues. This pattern of organizational growth was repeated in city after city as the epidemic found a place in smaller, more dispersed urban locales.

Although AIDS activist groups appeared to conform to traditional concepts of social movements, in which growth and transformation stem from spreading change in consciousness, the diffusion of AIDS activism followed the strange peregrinations of a communicable disease. Not only did the contexts of oppression—and the consciousnesses appropriate to these—shift, but science also exerted direct pressure on groups' self-conceptualization in the process. Where activists saw communities ripe for ideological transformation, epidemiologists saw collectivities linked through common behavior and a virus. Marxist ideas about mobilizing individuals by confronting them with the brute contradictions they lived was confused with the health-education idea that those who knew a person living (badly, of course) with AIDS would change their behavior. This muted but sadistic version of scare tactics seemed so intuitively correct that it went unchallenged— by educators, community organizations, and public health officials. Tireless people living with AIDS traveled far and wide—sometimes running themselves into the grave— to put a "face on AIDS," even though their courage contradicted the implicit logic of their acts: They were not scary, but heroic. Tragically, the tension within the meaning of living with AIDS—the truncated life's cautionary status in public health education versus the promise of survival that any life inspired among gay men—lent credence to the idea that AIDS had to be present before any real organizing could take place.

AIDS service organizations experienced the contradictory force of the cautionary and heroic figures of the person living with AIDS as an organizational battle between promoting prevention and advocating for those who were already sick. The Helms amendment (1988), which restricted the language and concepts that could be used in AIDS education funded by the government, combined with burgeoning caseloads of sicker, poorer people with AIDS, tipped the balance for agencies struggling to provide both education and care. Agencies' funding was at risk if they were too pro-sex, which in turned threatened the care of tens of thousands of people living with AIDS. Producing useful safe-sex advice seemed to directly threaten the well-being of those who were already sick. Given the impossibility of producing solid, scientific evaluations of safe-sex campaigns, especially radically designed ones, agencies were more visibly *doing something* when they coped with overwhelming caseloads. The idea that changes in sexual mores might eventually render care of the sick unnecessary slipped from view. Safe-sex organizing would always happen too late, would seem more like a punishment just short of death than a hope for life.

Though staffed by many former volunteers and agitators and characterized by gay-positive corporate cultures, the semiautonomous AIDS groups increasingly conformed to the structural expectations of their government and corporate benefactors, who saw AIDS groups as representatives of a community. But the actual communities whom the groups served and from which they emerged were almost immediately dissatisfied: By the mid-1980s, just as this first wave of activism stabilized into organizations, the next generation of activists, many self-identifying as PLWAs, were tremendously frustrated. This second wave criticized both the government and the ambivalently powerful AIDS organizations, the former for being obstructionist, the latter for being reformist.

Medical advances and public health policy also played a role in the growing rifts among AIDS activists. The general acceptance of HIV as pathogenic in AIDS and the massive Centers for Disease Control (CDC) campaign to promote testing fractured the second wave into two rather different groups: agitators concerned principally with treatment and funding issues, and groups that formed around the emerging identity of PLWA, concerned with quality of care, antidiscrimination, and self-help. Until the antibody test was widely available and *used*, organizers made little distinction between "activists" and "people living with AIDS"—there was no means of identifying who was infected with HIV, and no one would have known what such an identification would have meant if a test had existed. Activists individually thought of themselves as either very sick or not sick. Testing made it possible for individuals to discover whether they had HIV antibodies and made it clearer that there were significant numbers of non–gay male cases. Agencies understood their constituency to be changing; activists' concepts of the meaning and source of radical consciousness tracked closer to clinicians' descriptions of the progress of HIV. By the late 1980s, analysis of retrospective data showed that although infection was almost surely fatal, HIV was not nearly as rapidly debilitating as it had first seemed. The average time from infection to diagnosable AIDS symptoms—especially after standardization of prophylactic care for *Pneumocystis carinii* pneumonia, for years, the number-one cause of death among people with HIV—might be twelve years or even longer. And life span after AIDS diagnosis—a medical process increasingly complex because of the variety of opportunistic infections, cancers, and generalized markers of immune disfunction that could indicate AIDS—ranged from one to ten years, or longer in a small percentage of cases that should have been vigorously studied but were for some years treated as misdiagnoses. AIDS was transformed from a mystery ailment associated with rapid decline to death, into a loping, placid disease, ambiguously related to a retrovirus, a disease that could be managed with recalibrated existing treatments but whose long-term course could not (yet?) be stopped, even with synthetic antiretroviral agents.

The now-pervasive idea that some people had a greater personal investment in organizing *because* they were infected with a retrovirus did not emerge until 1986 or so. The abrupt shift in activists' sense of who was the true community affected by the epidemic was the effect of a scientific innovation: the antibody test that defined as one class of people those with a virus, whether they were symptomatic or not. In the 1960s and 1970s, black and then gay activists had painfully wrought an association between community and identity, identity and community. In the same way, serostatus and the extent of opportunistic infection (rather than "feeling sick") defined personal identity and thus several relationships to the epidemic, as if these were a natural association. The primary community was now understood to be the already-infected, and individuals' investment in activism was now viewed—whether to allege politicizing self-interest or righteous authentic experience—as a function of their serostatus. Seronegative gay men who worked for ASOs or public health agencies could now be held in contempt for "making a career" out of their brothers' misfortune. Straight women were largely exempt from criticism because their interests could be written into a larger cultural narrative of fag-haggery[8]—unless, of course, they raised women's issues. In that case, they suffered a fate like that of some lesbians, who, though longtime antihomophobia activists and advocates for improved care for lesbians and gay men, were accused of playing the gender card in the context of a disease that was not properly their own or were even accused of having "AIDS envy" when they tried to sustain political links with gay men through the plight of lesbians infected with HIV.

I return to these early years, the years before the antibody test was in use, to recall the early activists who were dead before *having the virus* took on identity status: These men and women, at least some of them, had different visions of solidarity, but because of their place in the spacetime of the epidemic, they are not counted as the original activist-seropositives. After the introduction of the test, those who had not died were presumed to be seronegative until they declared themselves otherwise. Although they had already fought hard, non-positives "after the test" were thought to be less able to understand the issues, which were increasingly narrowly defined as treatment and care, over and against prevention, broad-based community building, and health care activism. The initially serostatus-blind organizing articulated AIDS as a political issue first: Differences in strategies for confronting scientists, for demanding care and treatment, for changing sexual practices were *political* differences, not differences that arose from participants' serostatus. Only occasionally did people living with AIDS claim their illness as an identity-conveying difference—and rightly, when strategies were indifferent to their immediate situation. Activists who were diagnosed with AIDS were understood to represent a political condition as well as a medical one.

Most activists—regardless of their serostatus or their refusal to discover their serostatus—believed they should ensure the ongoing participation by people who were diagnosed with AIDS. This was often difficult, since, especially in the early years, those diagnosed with AIDS were usually fairly sick and did not necessarily have the energy for endless meetings. Anxious to maintain continuity in their leadership, some organizations may well have considered health status when hiring their first employees. Other groups dedicated a fixed number of positions on their boards of directors for seropositive individuals, who could work out their attendance and continuity for themselves. Setting board quotas and debating about whether to hire seropositive employees exacerbated the division along serostatus lines: AIDS groups were soon seen as being run by the worried well.

This reaction was strongest among gay men. There was much less division between women or injecting drug users of different serostatuses. Gay male seropositives tried to close ranks with seropositive women and drug injectors, but these latter groups as often as not preferred solidarity with their own racial, ethnic, or friendship groups. The National Association of People with AIDS and many local support groups succeeded in maintaining a space for diverse seropositive persons regardless of community of affiliation, but they accomplished this unity primarily by asserting a solid PLWA identity rather than by actually overcoming sexism, racism, homophobia, and so on.

The reactive formation of organizations or projects by and for seropositives, within or outside of AIDS groups, had the consequence of both privileging and marginalizing PLWA voices. This attention to negotiating the meaning and status of differences in serology and stage of illness had a dramatic and dire consequence for prevention work: Despite exhortations that seropositives should practice safe sex to avoid reinfection, most of the emerging organizations viewed safe sex as no longer relevant to seropositives. Perhaps these groups were trying to counter the government's tendency to put full responsibility for ensuring safe sex onto seropositives, a punitive idea of safe sex that meant seropositives should refrain entirely from sex in order not to infect anyone else. In the face of hysterical media campaigns about homicidal PLWAs (usually represented as gay men or prostitutes) infecting anyone and everyone, it was daunting to frame positive, radical safe-sex campaigns that did not seem complicit with admonitions to "just say no." Mainstream refusals to adopt condoms, compounded by the government's official advice to "choose carefully," made it virtually impossible to craft advice that was coherent for gay men, women, and the increasingly vilified "bisexual" male who allegedly connected them. Perhaps the reality that not everyone whom one knew to be infected was practicing safe sex was too hard to face. Maybe the as-yet-uninfected felt too guilty in their relief. Whatever the complex systemic and individual reasons, prevention activism was eclipsed by demands for improved treatment. Scrambling in the wake of the Helms amendment and faced with responding to more people with more-desperate needs, the large organizations put fewer resources and less attention into prevention than care. Only occasional projects (notably GMHC's safe-sex video shorts) from major agencies that had members from the earlier, more gay liberationist–inspired days were open to radical safe-sex work.

ACT UP emerged in 1987 with two points of contact with the community-based organizations: their common concern with treatment issues and with the vacuum in prevention education created by the Helms amendment and by the general drift away from future-oriented organizing of sexuality. In both contexts, ACT UP used highly sophisticated media-grabbing techniques: They rejected the more common New Left idea that demonstrating was about unmasking ideology or gaining a public voice in order to speak the Truth, which news reporters and their cameras would transparently reproduce. Despite their accusations of "lie!" ACT UP operated beyond any simple idea of a truth about AIDS.[9] They did not so much reject the idea of a truth as express a profound skepticism about the systems and processes through which scientific and political knowledge are produced. In their first five years, ACT UP members hit the books and demonstrated a stunning grasp of the quantifiable dimensions of the epidemic. They used facts and figures to bolster a moral argument. But they did not state the number of cases or the price of drugs, explain the economics of profit or the statistical problems in AZT trials, in order to—or not only in order to—correct the media. ACT UP demonstrated that ordinary people could understand the relevant science and demanded the acceptance of the *moral* truth juxtaposed to the numbers in the exquisite artistry of their posters and theatrical political actions. ACT UP went beyond McLuhan's proclamation that "the medium is the message," beyond even Jean Baudrillard's claim that the map precedes the territory. Their scientific acuity and dramatic staging produced a double helix in which science is a moral truth and morality is good science.

At first, ACT UP's efforts seemed like bizarre, undignified demonstrations: staging "die-ins," throwing fake blood on buildings occupied by researchers or government officials, soaking fake money in fake blood and raining it on Wall Street. ACT UP's style set it apart from groups operating from the traditional views that there is a central truth for social movements and that they are slow processes for transformation of individual consciousness and finally of the social order. Conventional activists viewed ACT UP as cynical, heavily tactical, too concerned with specific immediate problems, and too filled with the postmodern antipathy toward the grand theories of social change that might have helped them envision larger strategies.

In fact, most individual activists engaged in projects and actions that reflected both theories of activism. However, the differences between the two forms of activism, which held conflicting notions of how social change occurs and even of what social movement *is*, solidified in the organizations and policies that emerged in relation to these activisms. These concepts of change, and their contingent relationship to science and politics, were finally globalized as AIDS and AIDS activism. Grounded in the idea that people who have faced like conditions of oppression will share a collective consciousness, the community-based organization emblematized and resecured the civil collectivity it served. By contrast, although they refused the security of a liberatable consciousness, those who pursued discursive incursions tried to highlight the distribution and production of power. However well the two tactics worked, their limits revealed that both were incapable of fully understanding and changing all the problems associated with the epidemic. For example, community-based organizations do give aid and comfort to people who are rebuffed by the mainstream care systems; however, grounding politics in one identity, such as gay or PLWA, makes it difficult to adjudicate conflicts that arise along other dimensions of identity, such as black, poor, or female. Furthermore, by too starkly casting the villains—callous doctor or nurse, greedy researcher, homophobic or racist politician—identity-based politics obscured from critical analysis the ways in which even the most oppressed must nonetheless participate in the structures that oppress them.

Similarly, ACT UP's critical insight, as moments of shattering institutional façades, seemed to work only once; repetition in other places did not ensure that local activisms truly attended to the local conditions of power. Indeed, the "location" of ACT UP's interventions has often been *in discourse*, even if the actions themselves occur at a building taken to house the discourse's administrators. Whereas community-based organizations became semiblind to the power structures against which they had first constructed themselves, ACT UP lost its incisiveness when it ceased to realize that it had been the combination of mass support, solid documentation, and hard-hitting graphics, and not theatricality alone, that had disrupted scientific and moral logics.

All of these forms of political organizing have had international effects: Their strengths have enabled international activism to move swiftly, and their differences continue to produce conflicts—though sometimes in new forms—among types of AIDS activism internationally, between AIDS activism and gay activism, and among gay activists. Autonomous organizations like those that emerged in U.S. gay communities have served as the model for community-based programming in a wide variety of countries, even in places where they were the first NGO or in which there is no volunteer sector (WHO 1990). Similarly, the self-help-oriented PLWA movement spawned both local organizations and transnational networks. Carved out in the margins at international conferences on AIDS, "consumers" have become a significant presence in global research and policy development. The much-touted TASO (The AIDS Service Organization) in Uganda, a nearly exact replica of U.S. self-help groups, has prompted aid organizations concerned with other issues to also follow their model. Funding agencies and news reporters seem to like this form of community response, and local groups, anxious to gain money and visibility, have remade themselves to fit. Actual local impulses and desires are often lost in the mimesis of political action. For example, breast cancer organizing in the United States seems to have adopted the strategies of mainstream AIDS activism, but these strategies may have been adopted primarily because the media can register this model as "action" and report it. A once unrepresentable ailment has found an image by analogy: Pink ribbons now invoke a borrowed sympathy and signal political as well as memorial intent. We may never know whether this is the right style of politics.

Although less popular outside of Anglo-European countries, ACT UP and its most visible leaders moved from relative obscurity in the late 1980s to structural incorporation in the 1990s. Perceived as the leaders of a transnational opposition, colorful—or rather, black-clad—ACT UPers became required sources in televisual and printed news accounts about U.S. government AIDS policies. They became a force to be negotiated with at the annual International Conference on AIDS, the major performance space for their global visibility. This globalization of a particular image of opposition created several paradoxes as ACT UP's antigovernment rhetoric overtook its critique of science and policy. Other governments and international news sources could use ACT UP as a mouthpiece for their own anti-American sentiments. In other cases, both AIDS *and* the most vocal critics of AIDS policies could be seen as Yankee exports. This international prominence paradoxically lent more credibility to American activists' work at home, as if their local ACT UP groups and Third World nations necessarily shared the same goals.

The cultural criticism associated with late 1980s AIDS activism has also had a major impact on local organizing and global policy. This critical work has sometimes been attacked for misdirecting local U.S. activism; however, its surgical-strike interventions into several key areas of global policy have gone almost unnoticed. As a transnational professional language with a strong, reflexive multidisciplinary and political base, poststructural and social constructionist theories were each capable of insinuating new ideas about sexuality into global organizations that were struggling to be less colonialist. The strong association between cultural criticism and ACT UP made it hard for critics to see how poststructurally influenced forms of analysis had subtly but critically reframed international AIDS policy. Some Western critics of the cultural critiques admitted that postmodern tactics might have their place in hyper-industrialized countries, but they argued that such tactics were inapplicable in the developing world. This critique dovetailed with the official rejection by the governments of developing nations of feminism, gay liberation, and prostitute organizing. This conflation of ACT UP actions and poststructural cultural criticism romanticized Third World countries: Supposedly overwhelmed by the harsh practicalities of their physical environments or backward governments, countries outside the European and North American contexts were imaged as not needing the luxury of transnational or sexual politics. Envisioning an ACT UP in Dar es Salaam or a Queer Nation lodged within such extremely territorializing nations as Israel, Bosnia, or post-martial-law Taiwan taxed the Euro-American imagination. But local residents of these places know about

ACT UP and Queer Nation and are intrigued by these new, fractious politics and excited to find their own way to expose the contingency of the nation, established or emergent. To the extent that they were also post- or anti-colonialist, postpositivist theories of society and of social change were often more appealing to local activists than were traditional liberal modernist or Marxist approaches, which bore a legacy of imperialism.

I wanted to describe the first decade or so of AIDS activisms and their discontents as I witnessed and participated in them in order to create a pragmatic turn of mind before I take up what may at first seem like the abstract issue of the role of medical thinking in global AIDS representation and policy. In particular, I wanted to invoke the idea of activisms before The Name in order to suggest that AIDS is not a fixed thing, a natural phenomenon that necessarily engenders one response or another. Disease hits people in particular locations, but the concepts and responses that aggregate as AIDS inextricably reframe local experience. Both community-based (local) and discursive (translocal) forms of activism mean and do differently in different contexts. AIDS work interacts in complex ways with historically changing systems of medical knowledge and government power. The nexus of the global organizations that fund and direct policy and the media that represent the global epidemic to countries and the world forms a crucial space for how the epidemic will be conceptualized and handled in the years to come.

I have always argued that biomedical discourse and practices are key dimensions of global and local policies, though not in regular or straightforward ways. The traditional left and minoritizing approaches to resistance, which rely, respectively, on a belief in a fundamental, universal *class* consciousness and a fractional identity based in a shared history of oppression, are primarily concerned with the ideology and practices of the state. From these perspectives, the distribution of care and the conduct of science are primarily extensions of the state. These analyses of capital investment in medicine and of discrimination based on social attitudes are important, but they always underestimate the power of medical thoughtstyles to structure the terms through which bodies become visible as the locations of disease, of an epidemic. Political economy and civil rights claims treat bodies after they have emerged as visibilities—workers, blacks, queers. Medical thoughtstyles form at least part of the screen through which unarticulated masses of protoplasm pass on their way to becoming bodies of a certain type, in a certain place. Redressing current inadequacies in research and care is not as simple as determining which is more powerful, science or the state. We must instead describe how, *in the present case*, the state, science, and public media overlap, detach, and collide—and with what effects on the bodies we are trying to protect. Without a doubt, the United States had a crucial role in setting global trends in thinking about and handling AIDS, but the international and transnational formulations of the epidemic have also shaped the way the United States can represent its place to itself. In this volume, I try to make sense of the globalization of AIDS through an analysis of a handful of particularly exemplary cases in which different medical thoughtstyles collided to produce disastrous policy.

CHAPTER 2

From Colonial Medicine to World Health

In the late twentieth century, the meaning—or at least the face—of colonialism changed. Power no longer rested as obviously in the military primping and posturing of a small number of super nations. Though managed by the marginally international forces of the United Nations and militarism disguised as humanitarianism they represent, already-fragmented territories were torn apart by ethnic claims to nation status and by religious fundamentalist ambitions for theo-political rule. Multinational corporations and transnational trade pacts, though still largely controlled by long-enduring European and American powers, now dominate economies. A feral capitalism and the bloody wars within and between developing countries mask a new form of colonialism: former political rivals no longer compete on and for their own land but, rather, in and through other people's territory, envisioned as consumer markets and sources of cheap labor.

Despite revolutions and the expedient return of now oddly shaped countries, the management of health sustains poor countries' dependence on European and American superpowers, with their kinder, gentler faces: The health of people living in client states is still contingent on their previous, overt masters. Health policy operates both *inter*nationally, in the sense of cooperative relations within the old system of nations, and *trans*nationally, in

the sense of arching over, even defying geopolitical definitions. Even a brief exploration of international health
policy reveals the sobering disorder of the colonial legacy.

The WHO and to some extent the nongovernment,
health-related, nonprofit organizations functioning across
the former colonial powers exert continuous pressure on
the local health organizations of poorer countries. The
intricate relations among drug companies, governmental
and private medical research, and postcolonial governments also exert indirect pressure on the people who fall
under their overlapping jurisdictions. The bodies that connect these two pressure gradients are either guinea pigs
for questionable new health products or dumping grounds
for outmoded or illegal ones. As economic units, emergent nations may occasionally form markets, but only in-
directly: rich countries buy surplus medical supplies from
multinational drug companies, then offer them to poor
countries as foreign aid or as part of WHO supply programs, designed to supplement the minuscule per capita
amounts that developing economies can allot to medical
systems.

The gap between *trans*national diseases and *inter*national responses became a key factor in the successes and
failures of AIDS-prevention and care initiatives. On the
one hand, HIV's capacity to completely defeat national
borders and identities facilitated the development and linking of a new kind of NGO. AIDS activism became a sort
of global identity politics that created community based
on serostatus in a world where communities are more often
abstract structures than face-to-face relationships. But on
the other hand, international funding and policy-approval

processes impeded the consistent implementation of the recommendations of AIDS policy summits because any country could claim that its national security—or more commonly, its culture—was at risk. For example, gay men, lesbians, prostitutes, and people living with HIV have met numerous times and have forged a shared identity as the health disenfranchised, which partially overcame local differences in the symbolic meaning of their sexualities, commerce, and medical status. These activists, as representatives of people living with AIDS, helped persuade the WHO of the late 1980s to early 1990s to assist in prevention projects by urging member countries to decriminalize homosexuality and prostitution. But governments balked. The United States, a key financier of such meetings, refuses to adopt the recommendations of the very people sent as representatives of its own NGOs, men and women whose groups were the model for AIDS-related NGOs worldwide.

Because of its disjunct position, both *of* and *over* nations, the WHO is the most visible location of a policy machine in which the teeth on the gears do not match, and so the gears slip as they turn. Even when they momentarily catch and turn together, the movement is likely to produce bizarre results. For example, a form of health-policy analysis popular in the 1980s evaluated economic impact based on both the cost of an individual's treatment and the value to the nation of his or her "lost productivity." This model makes a certain amount of sense when one is examining costs across countries with similar economic infrastructures and in which people of comparable economic status are affected by a disease. But this method turns sinister when used to compare the costs to developed versus those to developing nations, especially when the disease so dramatically cuts across intranational class and rural-urban differences. Using this equation to compare the cost of AIDS treatment in, say, the United States versus that in Zaire, we would discover that during the crucial policy-making years of the late 1980s, the direct costs per individual case in the United States were about $20,000 a year, while the direct costs in Zaire were a mere few hundred dollars a year, mostly because there were no drugs or services for sale.

In the other dimension of analysis—labor lost to the gross national product (GNP)—losing the stereotypical U.S. gay yuppy lawyer at age thirty-five might deprive the U.S. economy of $1 million in lifetime salary; losing the stereotypical Zairean mine worker at the same age might deprive his country of only about $14,000 in lifetime salary. Just taking the cases of the United States and Zaire on their faces, most of us, if asked to guess, would think that a few lawyers lost here and there would probably be less devastating to the U.S. economy as a whole than the loss of even a small number of the critical workforce of miners would be to the Zairean economy as a whole. But of course, this kind of analysis, which is relatively insensitive to issues like worker replacement, job mobility, and sector differences in productivity, is not designed for moral nuance; it is intended to help global planners understand diseases' economic impact and how to allocate resources most efficiently. Some critics of global planning have pointed out the patent absurdity of even thinking in these terms about a transnational disease spread through behaviors largely ignored in economic planning. Activists, too, were slow to develop a comprehensive analysis of the problems of global planning, instead focusing on local resource allocation and the global effects of multinational drug companies. Until the late 1990s (with the exception of *Beneath the Equator* [1999], Richard Parker's seminal work on the World Bank's role in AIDS funding), activists had little to say about economic forecasting and planning processes, the global-economy equivalents of scientific research endeavors that ACT UP routinely targeted for criticism in the early 1990s. Well-researched analysis of these administrative practices reveals the basic logic on which global resources planning rests: the rich get health, and the poor are seen as expendable. In the end, statistical analyses of global health economics only provide an objective rationale for the stingy isolationism that keeps the lion's share of treatment resources in the United States. Instead of revealing how little it would cost rich countries to buy health and life for people in poor countries, such analyses reinforce the idea that poor countries are already lost to the epidemic. Economic analysis cannot help us recognize that AIDS *in* Africa is a symptom of black people's history of exclusion from global prosperity and economic dependency enforced by lack of control over either local or global resources. Grotesque comparisons of the sort I just outlined between the United States and Zaire reveal what global health activists already know: No matter how one looks at it, life—or rather, losing it—is cheap for all but the most privileged.

This form of analysis and its policy consequences does not always make sense even among developed countries, where medical philosophies and care delivery systems may radically differ, not only, and obviously, between East and West, but also between quasi-socialized systems and profit-driven systems, between systems that promote wellness and those that deal primarily in pathology. The goal set at the WHO International Conference on Primary Care held in 1978 in Alma-Ata, U.S.S.R., whose slogan was "Health for all by the year two thousand," confronts radically incommensurable needs, abilities to do research and to deliver medicine, and philosophies about the body's basic wellness or pathogenicity.

Perhaps a transnational health-monitoring body could meet the challenge of coordinating and mediating these conflicts and gaps. At least in the various modernist democratic political models we have inherited, there is some conviction that metanational groups can put aside the prejudices of international difference and determine what is "best for all." But ultimately, such ideas and programs are implemented in nation spaces, often directly through national governments. The WHO is still funded principally by the United States and wealthy European nations.[1] Thus, the colonial and imperialist relations that preceded it— between European nations and their former African colonies and between the United States and its Central and Latin American neighbors—are haphazardly but inevitably re-inscribed. Even in the noble effort to globalize basic human rights, the very concept of "world health" teeters ambiguously between a democratic ideal and a genocidal fantasy: Does it mean a world in which health is distributed, or one from which the unhealthy have been eliminated by any means necessary?

I want to suggest here that the problems in global policy are not always, and possibly are not even principally, issues of governmental relations. They may be less contingent on resource differences than at first seems so glaringly to be the case. Competing policies and misalignment of agency structures are importantly related to *different ways of imagining disease*, to the application of science in policy, and especially to the representation of those applications in media and public awareness campaigns. I want to suggest that the language and concepts used to articulate AIDS policy and to represent the epidemic to the world derive from two intertwined but nevertheless divergent medical thoughtstyles. One style, though deeply invested in its colonial history, is international, while the other, apparently divested of the idea of nation, is transnational. These two thoughtstyles are always both present in global and local conceptualizations of the epidemic, where they vie for narrative control. The first, which finds its images in tropical medicine, dominated the thinking of the WHO. The second, for which epidemiology provides the animating logic, dominated U.S. thinking about its epidemic, at least through the early 1990s, when "the face of AIDS" was said to have shifted toward "minority" populations and the spaces they were said to occupy (i.e., "the ghetto"). Because of U.S. scientific and political dominance, epidemiologic thinking caromed throughout AIDS medical research globally. As I will suggest later when I compare coverage of and papers presented at the Fourteenth International Conference on AIDS (2000, Durban), the epidemiological model still seems dominant, despite the representational shift toward the tropical model. The 1980s struggle between the two thoughtstyles belies science's view of itself as coherent and policy and media writers' belief that they can "apply" objective knowledge. Writers and policy makers became caught in the contradictions between the two ways of telling the story of AIDS. In the cases that follow here, we will see writers alternate between the narrative strategies available to them, not because they do not recognize or understand the underlying medical logics (although they may not) but because the bodies described sometimes outrun the stories that intend to secure a single meaning for their plight. The media and policy narration of the AIDS epidemic is a particularly spectacular example of the switching, drifting, patchwork use of supposedly disinvested descriptive frames, a tragic lesson in the extent to which medical knowledge is mediated in radically different ways, with geometrically increasing ill effects.

Tropical and Epidemiological Thought

At the risk of historical oversimplification, I want to detail two thoughtstyles that reflect the scientific concerns of Europe and the United States at the time of nineteenth- and early-twentieth-century urbanization and colonial expansion. Tropical thinking was concerned with the problems Europeans and Americans encountered in their distant occupations, reflecting both the reality and the fantasy of the colony. Tropical thinking was crucial to the development of certain modern concepts of disease; as Bruno Latour (1988) has shown, the displacement of the scientific laboratory from the academy to the field was crucial to the discovery of etiologic agents, in part because it enabled researchers to study diseases across a wide range of cases—a population—and in action. This resulted in the correlation of once only hypothetical disease agents with actual illness, finally establishing germ theory and the technology of vaccination. But equally, the late-nineteenth-century version of germ theory made sense because it was consistent with the political logic of invasion and occupation. Like much nineteenth-and early-twentieth-century social thought, colonialism operated through homology: the scientist's lab was not an organ of the state; rather, it sat in homologous relation, as the state, to the domain of disease, over which it held paternal control. Similarly, the colony of germs was homologously represented in a body or on an agar plate. Tropical medicine tried to predict where disease might be by analyzing the chain of homologous spaces—from the state to the agar plate—that were characterized by the telescoping structure of power relations.

Tropical medicine was feasible because colonial administrators believed that local diseases did not affect indigenous people in the same way they affected the European or American occupier. A tropical disease was understood to be proper to a place, to a *there*, but only to operate *as disease* when it afflicted people from *here*. Pathogens in a locale were recorded in medical history mainly when they appeared as disease in a colonist's body. Tropical disease was contained by virtue of already being *there*, in the "tropics." Critically, the very idea of tropical medicine rested on the ability to reliably separate an indigenous population, thought to be physically hearty but biologically inferior, from a colonizing population, believed to be biologically superior even though subject to the tropical illnesses. Tropical medicine thus grew out of and supported the idea that a First World body is the proper gauge of health; the Third World is the location of disease, even though its occupants are not properly the subjects of tropical medicine. Tropical medicine points to a presupposed map and hierarchy of bodies. Only Europeans are subjects in tropical accounts, and not in relation to disease but in relation to a prior presumption about "being from here."

Coloniality centered on anxieties about being—and compulsions to *be—in proximity* to the primitive. In tropical medicine, these concerns inspired an interest in natural immunity, the capacity to live in proximity to germs that appeared to characterize the colonized. Through the homology of possession, colonial inhabitation soon had the fantasy of acquiring not only the land and its people but also immunity, and in advance: Immunization could provide the means of safe colonial occupation. Obsessed with the ailments that seized the European in the tropics, disease was described in melodramatic terms, as the monster inside the domestic space, the evil endemic to the colony. Narrating disease according to the melodramatic formula also complexly gendered the personae of the tropical tableaux. The fantasy of acquiring immunity—of having the natives' immunity, even their blood, enter one's body—might have feminized the colonist. Achieving immunity might also have erased the difference that susceptibility to disease marked. But tropical thinking was confident of its implicit geographical scheme, in which the First World is always superior to the Third World. The quest for immunity sustained the hierarchical difference between the colonized, immune body and the colonizing, immunizable body. Reversing the culturally legible fear of being penetrated by alien germs, the (masculine) colonist turned his weakness into a tale of fearlessness. The vaccinated colonizing body could safely live in close proximity to, by colonizing the very immunity of, the colonized body that is conceived as being "naturally" close to disease.

The melodramatic narrative sensibility of tropical thinking produced a family drama in which incursion into the constructed domestic space of the colony was accompanied by nostalgia for "going home." The diasporal drama of displacement and return meant that even if the colonist could not always get well, he could always go home. The colonist's ailing body was heroic, not the victim of dislocation but the most intimate site of domesticating the tropics. Both the sick European body and the body of the researcher or physician participated in this drama: A physician might go to the colony to treat afflicted European bodies, or he or she might go to treat natives Europeanized by imported, "civilized" diseases. Tiptoeing forgetfully in the tracks of European and American generals, who sometimes carried out their genocidal fantasies by medical means, researching physicians would eventually claim a victory for world health by eradicating from the Third World the very smallpox that Europeans had imported. But the disease suffered a politically significant downgrading. Smallpox, originally a "civilized" disease, was exported to the tropics at the same time that it was being eliminated in Europe and was rewritten as endemic to the tropics; the disease went native, becoming a mark of Third World biological inferiority instead of a badge of colonial violation.

In order to curb the reintroduction of smallpox, world health planners engaged in a cartographic practice that, while largely keeping smallpox out of Europe, also established a general procedure that has had dire political consequences, not the least of which is the insult of further penalizing those unable to resist the infliction of Europeans' biological detritus. Tropical thinking superimposed its value-ladden here/there view of civilized and noncivilized space on the geomedical and thus fixed disease in place. These diseases, which are regulated by national medical establishments but which are also regulating—of those who have them—doubly but asymmetrically marked space: Where there are tropical diseases, there must be lack of civilization (tropics), and where there is civilization there must be lack of (tropical) disease. These tautological definitions of disease and place were laminated onto one another, forming a thick map of ailing bodies that also projected solutions. Tropical medicine now had at its disposal two means to achieve domestication unhampered by disease: to immunize the colonizers before they left Europe, and to police the health of those who returned. In order to ensure that tropical disease did not slip unnoticed into Europe in the unnaturally and naturally immune bodies of returning colonials and immigrating natives, a worldwide immunization scheme was conjured up. Fundamental to the plan for eradicating smallpox was a new requirement that one carry immunization stamps. But even immunization had double meaning, depending on the origin of the body bearing the vaccine's scar. Smallpox vaccination now marked two modes of *becoming* civilized; even this leveling of susceptibility sustained the colonizer/colonized structure. The scar left by the vaccination marked either the body prepared to admit itself to the master culture or the body protecting itself against the return of those who had survived the colonial occupation. This is the global precursor to the much-criticized but intransigent duality in AIDS thinking: The colonial subject (or homosexual or prostitute) is presumed to be infectious, while the colonizer (or "mainstream" person) is presumed open to infection.

Epidemiology, tropical thinking's urban cousin, was also concerned to mark differences, but within the teeming metropole. Far from viewing the body in Europe as essentially clean, epidemiology believed that germs were anywhere and everywhere, even if they were not (yet) causing problems. Epidemiology told the story of pathogens, not of bodies or places. Through its new form of reasoning, especially emerging statistical technologies, the separation of the germ's story from the body allowed epidemiology to declare "disease" from some but not all conjunctures of body and pathogen.

Epidemiology operated from an apparently simple definition: An epidemic is more cases of a disease than expected. Declaring an epidemic depends on the expectation that in its perpetual movement, pathology would become visible against a background state of health. These migratory sites of pathology could at any time be linked through "vectors," the traces of movement outward from a center. Each new locale became a new center capable of projecting its links to further peripheries, which in turn became new centers. Unlike tropical thinking's richly and melodramatically narrated story of the diasporal movement of disease, epidemiology's vector patterns were multidirectional, coolly geometrical, antinarrative, and figural. Each new movement defeated any sense of return, for disease always marched *forward*, even if in several directions at once.

Tropical thinking held two kinds of body in constant view: those from "here" and those "we" might encounter "there." Epidemiology was only interested in bodies once they were affected by and had become perpetrators of pathology. Each body of epidemiology is both "sick" and a reservoir or carrier, a distinct moment of and linkage in the larger network of disease. Epidemiology was concerned not so much with detailing or treating the diseases that befell the European body in a place but with visualizing— often with graphs—the march of bodies that made visible the temporal sequence called "epidemic." The body fighting disease was not heroic; rather it was a mere example of what happens before other medical disciplines break the chain of vectorality discovered by epidemiology.

Tropical medicine could predict disease because it already knew where disease was and who could fall sick. Refusing, for the most part, tropical medicine's comforting map of the world, epidemiology had to describe the space of disease and indicate the bodies most likely to harbor or transport it, simultaneously describing a place and predicting a sequence, creating a space-time for epidemic disease. Bereft of a stable *place* of pathology, epidemiology had to constantly construct and correlate populations and subpopulations in order to make epidemics visible—hence its reliance on the descriptive and predictive technologies of surveillance and sentinel studies.[2] Only the disease detectives, according to epidemiological thinking, have the power to visualize the natural history of germs' vectoral movement.

The subjects and diseases always changed (different risk groups for different diseases); the absolute center of an epidemic perpetually shifted. This mobility of place and reclassification of bodies destabilized tropical medicine's idea that disease belonged to certain bodies, and the fantasies of immunity that went with it. Epidemiologists merely packed their tents and moved on to a new epicenter, secure in their capacity to trace the movements of new symptoms through new configurations of bodies. Epidemiology not only invented the vectors and subjects of disease but also situated itself as the optimal place from which to observe the progress of a disease. In principle, epidemiology made no a priori distinctions about bodies or places. In theory, any body could be a vector. Epidemiology's job was to discover which bodies actually connected the hot spots of disease outbreak. Disease, rather than the bodies where it may take place, was conceived as the real bedrock of an epidemic.

Whereas tropical medicine grounded itself in stable ideas of place and of hierarchies of bodies, epidemiology wrote itself in relation to a background definition of health. If the colonial homology could mask the medical crimes of transporting disease *to* the colony, epidemiology could hide the crimes of class-tiered health care delivery by naturalizing the background definition of health used to mark an epidemic: *Health* was the natural state of the middle class. Though both medical logics tended to protect the same people, their health was in jeopardy for different reasons. The (masculine) colonist got sick because he was in the tropics. The middle class envisioned by epidemiology was in danger because disease refused to respect the natural but unspatialized boundaries of health. Thus, epidemics would be noticed largely if and when they threatened the middle class, and later, as with polio in the 1950s, when they were proper to the middle class. Epidemiology reversed tropical medicine's concern with who might fall sick by removing disease from the natural environment (the native's body constituting part of Nature) and placing it in the body of the displaced Other. Instead of seeing tropical inhabitants as more or less immune to the diseases that surround them, epidemiology saw the indigines as mobile locations of disease: reservoirs, carriers. Poverty was no longer natural and was thus no longer spatially limited; now, it threatened the middle classes with contagion.

Epidemiology defined the boundaries of a disease by constituting an imagined community ("risk group") described through vectors that epidemiology presented as though discovered. Disease may radiate out from a place— an epicenter—but it was rarely proper to that place. An epicenter is, by definition, unstable and uncontained. Epidemic disease must be confined and policed. The concern for *public health* entailed a very different notion of the domestic. Epidemiology conceived the domestic not as a space of delicate coexistence, as in the intricate tropical homologies centering on immunity, but, rather, as nonarticulated space, the smooth space where disease has not penetrated, the space to be protected by exposing—publicizing—the mobile space of disease. Thus, epidemiology seeks eradication of disease, either through spreading cures or through eliminating vectors, that is, through isolating the disease within the vectoral bodies and by separating infected from healthy bodies.

For epidemiology, the first line of defense is to seal off the disease within the afflicted body, to cure it, or at least to prevent its migration outside that body. For AIDS, epidemiology tends to understand curative drugs and condoms as a means of containment, of keeping HIV *in* the infected cell or infected body rather than highlighting their "positive" capacity of keeping HIV *out* of the uninfected cell or body. In or out: These are not as reciprocal as they seem, for they signal life and death—or at least a life maintained by toxic regimes—for actual people who are, for epidemiology, mere reservoirs. Far from being opposite sides of one coin, "in" and "out" signify kinds of space. The infected site is articulated, rough; it is the cell or body that is the object of scrutiny, and policing it is presumed to keep disease from going to nonarticulated, smooth space *elsewhere*.

Only in the absence of these first-order containment possibilities is the second line of defense invoked: cordoning off the actual bodies affected. In quarantine, epidemiology appears to converge with tropical medicine's ideas of fixed place; epidemiology risks collapsing the space of disease and the space of the body.[3] Insofar as a quarantine ward or camp is the location of disease contained, it is like an Othered tropic. However, in tropical thinking, the tropical body and tropical space are equivalent; a body's relation to tropical disease distinguishes *this* space from the European center. The quarantine ward or camp temporarily freezes body-disease and space within a temporal flow. These bodies *become* diseased and are territorialized not because there is some preexisting affinity between these bodies and a space but because they have come to harbor pathogens; they are themselves moments in the space-time of disease. Thus, the germ defines the quarantine space. The bodies are only incidentally captured there as unfortunate (but nonetheless reviled) vehicles. Because epidemiology is concerned with containing germs' vectorial movement in order to prevent disease vectors from simply going ballistic (in the technical sense of going off a straight path), epidemiological thinking holds that the infected bodies must be held in place-time, causing an intensification of disease in that spot—like a hot tropic— but only because *un*natural containment has *set in*.

Like Marx's promise of a new "Time after History," epidemiology's promise was of a new history of the healthy body on the other side of the natural time of the diseases the discipline catalogs and represents. At its political zenith, in the mid-twentieth century, epidemiology was conceived as the central line of defense against disease: Clinical, administrative, and research enterprises responded to epidemiology's fateful call, making disease outbreaks real. But these partners threatened epidemiology at the same time that they served it: They wanted to destroy disease, dissipating the object of the epidemiologic gaze. Thus, epidemiology secretly demanded of a disease that it persist, at least long enough to be registered as successive epidemics. Even after the sister disciplines set about their disease-destroying work, it was difficult for epidemiology to release its grip on the germs it had lovingly graphed. In order to continue writing the natural history of a disease—its history before being controlled—epidemiology needed to keep some of the ailing bodies for itself. In order to show the truth of its own history, epidemiology was continually tempted to let the disease run its course. Though there are plenty of good reasons to conduct placebo-controlled studies of treatment, the practice sometimes feeds this secret lust of epidemiology.[4]

Although I have intentionally overdrawn the differences between two medical disciplines that often cooperate quite happily, I think the characterization of the underlying thoughtstyles is borne out in their practices. In the spring of 2000, I attended a conference on travel medicine. The conference was packed with the latest information on what ailments travelers, especially travelers to exotic places, are likely to get. Hardly a presentation went by without giant pictures of parasitic worms crawling under someone's skin or across the sclera of an eyeball. So often were we treated to huge magnified versions of exquisite but deadly parasite-carrying bugs that I doubt anyone left with any lingering doubt about the physiology of the mosquito. In short, the largely tropical-medicine focus of the conference was made vivid in the gleeful researchers' wild travel tales and graphic slides, both of their exotic destinations and of the creepy things they found there, the weirder the better.

This was all quite strange to me, because I have spent many equally happy hours attending medical conferences dominated by epidemiologists. And indeed, I did attend one of the few presentations that offered a narrative different from that of wild and weird experiences of tropical clinicians in odd places. Because the conference was located in New Mexico, one of the epicenters of the recent outbreaks of *Hantavirus*-related illness, there was a small session on the epidemiology of the newly emergent disease syndrome associated with the rodent-borne virus. Much to the boredom of my colleagues, who were socialized in tropical medicine rather than epidemiology, the researcher told of the shock and surprise of encountering some of the first cases. He described himself as baffled by the sudden death of a young patient and by the quick decline and death of index patient's wife. Instead of pictures of icky worms and elegant mosquitoes, this researcher had time charts and maps to show us when and where cases had been discovered. There was also a sort of family-tree chart, based on genetic research, showing the relationship between *Hantavirus* and several similar viruses in Asia and Europe. The story here was of detection: how the epidemiologists and clinicians figured out what had caused the unexpected rapid deaths. While I was intrigued by the complexity of tracking variant viral strains and of ascertaining how disease had moved from one place to another, I have no idea what a *Hantavirus* looks like, nor do I have any idea whether the reservation American Indians he had treated lived in mud cliff dwellings or in desert mansions.

A casual comparison of introductory epidemiology texts and tropical medicine texts reinforces the basic distinction here. Tropical medicine texts, almost universally decorated with a giant picture of a mosquito, recount the traveling history of the discipline. Born of Europeans' forays into warmer climes—eventually culturally constructed as "tropics"—the discipline balanced the allure of the weird and foreign with the physician's call to help the ailing. Contemporary textbooks show no anxiety about the differences in disease translocation that postmodern transportation has brought about, nor does the miniaturization of etiology agents (from bugs to microbes) seem to disrupt the fundamentally secure self-conception that tropical medicine has a scientific role even if there really are no tropics left "out there." If anything, the speed of disease movement seems to give tropical medicine more work, rather than less: the tropics are now everywhere.

By contrast, the epidemiology texts are torn, not knowing whether they are a method or a science, a poor stepchild to real science and real medicine or the interdisciplinary nexus of both. Consistent with my characterization here, epidemiology seems never to know its *place* until it is smack in the middle of tracking down a disease. Although statistical forecast is increasingly possible and a domain of epidemiology, the discipline seems always to dwell in its heroic past: Because the need for epidemiology evaporates as soon as it solves a disease problem, the texts must insistently reinforce the idea that epidemiology is central in the fight against disease.

Thus, I want to go on to lay out in detail the ways in which the two thoughtstyles provide importantly different ways to tell a medical story. Epidemiological narrative is most visible as it constructs movement, tropical narrative as it constructs place. How we read AIDS stories composed from these two forms of medical narration depends in part on how long we listen. The epidemiologic framing of AIDS seems in the moment to collapse into the tropical narrative, but then it recovers its explanatory power and moves on. Each account also varies with spatial positioning. From the local perspective, the epidemic *among* heterosexuals is vectorial, but from the global perspective, HIV's *arrival in* the body of a homosexual is diasporal. Let me graphically summarize the differences between the two thoughtstyles:

Tropical Thinking	Epidemiological Thinking
Argues through homology	Argues through metynomic production of statisical correlation
Is obsessed with proximity	Is obsessed with transfer, between bodies or disease pools
Always visualizes bodies in the colonial map	Abstracts bodies in data
Uses melodramatic narrative	Uses detective narrative
Sees disease "there"	Sees disease everywhere
Spatializes	Temporalizes
Is diasporal	Is vectorial
Defines bodies in advance and in relation to their original space	Defines and redefines bodies through categories related to disease
Considers all bodies meaningful	Acknowledges no meaning for bodies beyond their relation to a succession of diseases
Maps	Simulates
Presents immunity as the solution	Presents cure, breaking vectorial links as solutions
Is confounded when bodies "go native"—may allow for vectoriality	Is confounded by employing fragmentary descriptions of previous diseases—may resort to tropical maps

These two schemes envisioned different maps of world health, which in turn, had two effects on the first decade of strategies for managing the HIV pandemic, one quite literal and the other representational. Whereas the administration of global health funding occurred largely through a model related to the tropical image of the world, HIV and related disease surveillance literally employed epidemiology. During the crucial first decade of the epidemic, this science was produced and administered through an aberrant WHO branch called the Global Programme on AIDS (GPA).[5] Until the reorganization of HIV-related programs under the new UNAIDS project, the GPA generated scientific data and proposed policy based on one concept of disease, while the WHO attempted to effect and fund AIDS policy and programs based on another. Predictably enough, participant countries were often hostile to the programs designed by the GPA, and some of the most powerful funding countries refused to adopt GPA policy guidelines. As I noted earlier, the United States never took up the call to decriminalize homosexuality and prostitution proposed by the very project it had funded and promoted. I will elaborate this double mapping in chapter 3, "Official Maps."

The second level of effect concerns popular representation of the epidemic. Explanations of AIDS in newspapers, pamphlets, and books aimed at general readers vacillated between the accounts that the two different ways of narrating the epidemic make possible. Thus, a wide and contradictory set of stereotyped ideas about the epidemic and those it affects gained credibility through the invocation of either or both medical thoughtstyles. The thoughtstyles amounted to scientific citations for more wildly fictional accounts: Any cultural stereotype or political idea that could be recirculated or challenged by this association with science had far greater power than a stereotype that stood on its own. Thus, the way the story of AIDS is told has a potentially great effect on the acceptability of policies that are promoted within that story's narrative reach. To the extent that these two major scientific thought-styles framed representations of the epidemic, there were competing ways of claiming the mantle of neutrality that invoking science affords. The last half of this book works through a series of cases of this clash.

CHAPTER 3

Official Maps

A deeply spatial understanding of disease echoes in the WHO's division of the world into six administrative regions, a division that, as I will show, simultaneously naturalizes the designated units and largely cedes to individual nations political power within them. Because funds come from developed countries and—with the most delicate of strings—go to countries the West is interested in developing, the WHO continues to be in a tricky position: It must take care neither to offend the donor countries nor to make policies that are unpalatable to the client states. The WHO's role in global management has become increasingly daunting as local feelings about national identity have changed. Transnational capital has made the identities of industrialized nations an impediment to their global economic survival (think of the North American Free Trade Agreement [NAFTA] or the European Economic Community), while, in developing countries, the increasing conflation of religious or ethnic identity with national identity has given patriotism the feel of zealotry. National identities only seem to matter most to those who have no other form of global capital.

Established in the wake of European and American colonial and imperialist forays, the WHO regions reflect the unconscious of a particular historical epoch, the moral vision of the world that former colonial powers hoped to bring about. Perhaps not surprisingly, the entire Western

Hemisphere is a single region—the Pan American Health Organization (PAHO)—with its head offices in Washington, D.C. The nineteenth- and twentieth-century hemispheric isolationism, which simultaneously ensured U.S. domination over the Latin American countries and prevented Europeans from commenting much on the fact, is reproduced in the kinds of policies and programs PAHO engaged in prior to the HIV pandemic. Diseases lay in the *south*. For example, PAHO's first major report on the epidemic contained little on the United States except to offer northern solutions for problems the books defined as "different," almost tropical.

Europe and the British Isles make up a second region, although there is usually little participation from Great Britain, which, though home to colonial subjects, has withdrawn from the circumglobal empire it once created. Although U.K.-based NGOs have been active in Third World health projects, their enthusiastic volunteerism does not quite overcome the national responsibility Britain bears for the deplorable economic state of many of its former colonies. Britain also refuses to participate with its European neighbors, themselves reconfigured several times in the twentieth century. Much of Europe has now banded together in order to act *collectively* in their relations to the vast colonial territories of Africa that several nations once differentially administered and that still have the names— or at least the borders—that intra-European competition produced as trophies. In the context of the AIDS epidemic, and corresponding in time to the move toward an economically united Europe, the European group has been the region most effective at developing HIV-related anti-discrimination policy. Using the emerging European Community's governing bodies, which partially map the space the WHO defines as a health region, countries have brought pressure to bear on one another to promote more humanitarian care for people with AIDS, to support local organizing, and to develop cooperative projects in the Third World, especially with African countries. In the face of a disease that so poignantly defies nationality, European countries' invocation of human rights enables them to relinquish some control over national health policy, muting the political effects of national borders without challenging formal national sovereignty. Nevertheless, their *collective* relationship to their former client states in Africa has reinscribed a more general Eurocentrism in the face of an Other who is more different from Europeans than Europeans are from each other.

Asia and the Pacific are divided into two regions: Much of Asia and Australia and most of the Pacific Rim islands make up the Western Pacific region, and Mongolia, the Indian Subcontinent, and some of the Southeast Asian islands make up the Southeast Asia region. With the spectacular exception of research on Thailand's vast sex trade, there was little regional or national effort by the WHO to deal with AIDS in the Southeast Asia region in the 1980s. The 1990s shift to addressing AIDS "in Asia" occurred in the context of resurgent nationalism and religious fundamentalism. Whereas the rubric of region afforded Europe a means of blurring national distinctions in order to embrace the exigencies of a global pandemic, subsuming nation to region in Asia has produced an oppositional stance toward the West: The rhetoric of "Asian values" demanded that Westerners make good on their promises of cultural sensitivity. Once-disparate cultures now had a new rhetorical umbrella under which they could unite against Western ideas, including the concept of human rights invoked in open-border and antidiscrimination policies and the concept of individual autonomy—control over one's body—implicit in safe-sex education and proposals to decriminalize homosexuality and prostitution.

To some extent, health officials from these two regions perceive AIDS and AIDS-prevention advice to be intrinsically connected to sexualities that have emerged as an effect of the colonial legacy. Sex tourism, the proliferation of sexual discussion, and the representations that seemed necessary to promoting safe sex were each seen as resting on European and American concepts of sexuality. Although colonial management did have enormous effects on local sexualities, postcolonial rhetoric that purports to return to pre–colonial era cultural norms is often as puritanical—even explicitly Christian—as the European and American moralities their "return to" Asian values is meant to reject. Implicitly setting up an opposition between a rich traditional sexuality and an impoverished Americanized or Europeanized one devoid of meaning, several governments criticized condoms—the emblem of safe sex—as a cultural-imperialist tool.[1] An Indian campaign mobilized the then-current nationalist tendency to reconstruct a precolonial classicism as the true national culture. The lushly illustrated campaign first associated condoms with an alien culture in which sexual pluralism required promiscuity, and then proposed an alternative form of safe sex: the *Kama-sutra*. This practice, which Westerners view as the ultimate form of sexual experimentation, became a new kind of monogamy more exciting than the possibilities for partner change that the condom was said to afford: "Many positions with one, better than one position with many" (WHO 1993, 3).

The Western Pacific region deserves additional comment, because in a later section of this book, I will consider the failure to pursue HIV prevention there. This region lumps together *developing* nations with Japan and the largely Anglo (though multicultural)[2] Australia. Past WHO programs in this region mimicked the Europe-Africa structure, confounding colonial relations and races: (White) Australia inherited responsibility for the colonial ambitions of England, for which it once existed as a forced-labor colony, but Japan, as racial Other to the West, was frequently overlooked as a long-standing imperialist force within the region. As in the Southeast Asia region, neither individual countries nor the WHO took much interest in the possibility that AIDS might finally arrive in the region's developing countries. Australian safe-sex campaigns, some of the world's best for gay men, floundered when addressing aboriginal concerns. The case of an aboriginal nurse who rode her bike among aboriginal communities is an example of the disconnect between the GPA's borderless epidemiologic model and the nation-bound, client-state model of the larger WHO: Although she presented papers on her work at several GPA conferences and was touted as an exemplar of local response, she was never properly funded by the Australian government or the WHO, nor was her program systematically replicated elsewhere.

Japan and Australia came to occupy strange roles in the epidemic: As a *nation*, Japan, hyperindustrialized and by reputation sexually perverted, would appear to need exhaustive HIV education along the lines of that employed in the United States. But prevention education had, by the mid-1980s, boiled down to promoting condom use, and Japan's couples were already ranked first among nations as measured by condom use. It was difficult to imagine how to make the need for condoms seem like bad news.[3] Condoms had arrived in Japan *too soon* to take on the negative association of promiscuity that went with being the universal signifier of safe sex. But as a result, the highly aesthetic Japanese condoms posed a serious challenge to the U.S. product, even though the culture of male acceptance that ensured high levels of condom use in Japan failed to take hold in the United States. Australia, too, fought to make its product available elsewhere, and by the end of the 1980s, it listed its rough and tough Ansell condom among its most popular exports.

In the 1980s, Japan emerged as an economic and to some extent cultural competitor to the United States; during the same period, Australia tried to mute its Anglo heritage and to identify with its Asian neighbors. Ironically, Australia's model responsiveness to its epidemic—whose epidemiologic profile is virtually identical to the disease's initial years in the United States—only further widened the political gap between itself and the Asian nations, which were not very enthusiastic about including Australia in the broadened cultural category "Asians." Their mutual pasts as British colonies not withstanding, Australia had difficulty writing itself into an Asia, however culturally and politically fragmented, that was simultaneously reconstructing for itself a history of *continuous* cultural solidarity. The "Asian Values" asserted by national leaders were antithetical to the implicitly humanist multicultural Australian state, which viewed itself as the zenith of liberal pluralism and social welfare. The ambivalent cultural and economic relationship between Australia and its regional siblings was encapsulated in a late-1980s safe-sex campaign: Apparently directed toward Anglo-Australian travelers, one ad featured a Quantus jet sporting a condom, though it was uncertain whether such prophylaxis would contain the advanced epidemic within Australia or prevent tourists from bringing more back from elsewhere.

The fifth and sixth regions are Africa (in fact, subsaharan Africa) and the Eastern Mediterranean, which includes North Africa. The Eastern Mediterranean region pretends to cover a geographic region, but it actually corresponds to religious history, encompassing the nations that are the strongholds of Islam. These nations insisted, until well into the 1990s, that the austerity their religious commitments demanded served as a virtual barrier against HIV.

The idea and administrative use of regions implicitly insisted that the designated spaces should correspond to features of natural geography, as encompassed in ideas like hemispheres or continents. But whereas PAHO, Europe, and Africa—the West—are each comprised of roughly contiguous countries, Southeast Asia, the Eastern Mediterranean, and the Western Pacific each have marooned segments; the Southeast Asia region looks more like territorial islands than island territories. The human sociopolitical patterns that reinforced the apparent naturalness of the regions lent an air of destiny to the colonial structure that remained as a shadow in the place-names suppressed in favor of the regional designations. Like the very geology underlying the shifting details of geography, changes in national territories after colonialism have never forced the remapping of WHO regions. Rarely have countries been reassigned, nor have the regions been reconceptualized to meet changes in the health status or in the needs of countries' citizenry. Any similarities that exist in the patterns of health and disease that occur within a region are due to the combined history of a germs' favorite environment and accidents of geopolitics, not to the cultural affinities now used to justify the regions. The very idea of regions has been slow to change, and the WHO continues to be simultaneously a disinterested global administrator and a covert stablizer of those geopolitical relations. Health continues to be administered on a regional basis.

From Regions to Patterns: Mapping AIDS

These strange geographic compromises in an increasingly variable political context did not match the image of the world at risk from HIV held by U.S. public health officials, who first joined the WHO with the hope of globalizing America's hard-won lessons about AIDS. Under the direction of an epidemiologically oriented American (the late Jonathan Mann) with experience within the U.S. public health system, the GPA adopted a different mapping of the world, one importantly (but not completely coherently) linked to epidemiologic understandings of the disease writ large. The new GPA rejected preexisting ideas of the world's geopolitical composition—or used them only when hard data were unavailable—and replaced regions with *patterns* that purported to describe characteristic interactions among categories of invariable human sexual behavior. However, these patterns were grafted back into geopolitical stereotypes once the distinctiveness of the patterns failed to hold up. Instead of recognizing the plasticity of human sexual behavior, the patterns used cultural stereotypes to explain variations away.

The shift in nomenclature from "regions" to "patterns" echoed the more subtle shift away from a conceptualization of the *place* of disease from one that naturalized geography to one that simulated statistical distribution. Displacing the deeply inscribed geography of the regional system, the GPA proposed a *syndrome-specific* system, broadly dividing the world into physically contiguous but *temporally* conceived "patterns" that were numbered, not coincidentally, according to the rough order—that is, time sequence—in which epidemiologists had identified the global "emergence" of densities of cases up to about 1984. Pattern One, commonly called "AIDS," refers to places characterized by the gender-exclusive category of intercourse between men. Pattern Two, or what is now usually called "African AIDS," refers to places where intercourse between people of "opposite" genders appears to account for most cases of transmission. Pattern Three, the initially blank space of Asia where "AIDS arrived late," was defined through the absence of cases.

The shift from a complicated system defined by geopolitical regions and nations to a flatter, simpler map related to incidence probability obscured the fact that each *pattern* was actually defined using different criteria. Though cast in the general temporal sequence secured by emphasizing epidemiologic thinking, each pattern continued to tautologically reconstitute the criterion that had originally defined it. WHO could not abandon its regions to syndrome-specific nomenclatures. Who would fund attention to them? How would a quasi parliament of interested parties function? Who would be the object of policy implementation or censure? Whatever its flaws, the regional system allowed for geopolitical interconnection; thus, the regional and pattern schemes had to coexist. Whereas the *administrative* map, used to allocate resources, related to colonial notions of geography, the GPA's predictive map referred to spaces supposedly defined by transmission routes.

This coexistence created an institutional discourse that afforded broad possibilities when the media explained AIDS to the world. The official story forged from this internally incoherent institutional amalgam allowed for two kinds of story:

> Researchers believe that the virus was present in isolated population groups years before the epidemic began. Then the situation changed: people moved more often and travelled more; they settled in big cities; and

lifestyles changed, including patterns of sexual behaviour.
It became easier for HIV to spread, through sexual
intercourse and contaminated blood. As the virus spread,
the isolated disease already existing became a new
epidemic. (WHO 1989a, 6)

This now-commonplace account holds in tension in-
compatible ideas about disease and its translocation. Criss-
crossing temporal and geographic tropes, the account
vacillates between the *story* of a virus and a *description* of
bodies who might disperse it. "The virus" is described as
first lodging in a timeless and immobile *place:* grounded
in an "isolated population" until modernity stepped in to
inscribe time and a mania for travel. "Then," people began to move and change, carrying with them the dangerous
combination of their new sexual practices and their contaminated blood. Miraculously (inevitably?), an epidemic
ensued. Modernity catapulted the virus, which had once
lived peacefully among unnamed "population groups,"
into an epidemic of history-changing proportions. The
story completely naturalizes the idea that it was denation-
alized bodies—not corporate and state blood-banking
practices—that first dispersed HIV (Kramer 1993; Fleming 1988). Following this pattern, the Taiwanese account
(to which I will turn below) cannot register what it knows
about its own epidemic. Though a "transiting" American
homosexual is cited as the first known case of AIDS in
Taiwan (in 1984), infected blood products had beaten
him there. The then-new antibody test was not widely in
use, and no one could have known that transfusion recipients throughout the island had already been infected
with HIV. The Asian nations, at first unwitting and later re-

luctant recipients of poorly screened or unscreened blood, only registered their epidemics when travelers with AIDS were visible in their midst. The American in Taiwan was visible not, as the official travelogue story suggests, because he disembarked to begin a frenzied crusade to infect locals but because he was so sick he had to be rushed to the hospital.

The sketchy official account is like an Escher drawing: a template that allows a plethora of more-detailed versions of the story to transmute one into another. The central role of the migratory body is anonymous, allowing reporters and international health-policy analysts to enliven their accounts with "real people." Almost *anyone* could be implicated as the problematic mobile body. A Canadian airline steward or a jet-setting gay tourist, an African truck driver or the rural woman who sells him sex on the edges of the city, a male migrant laborer who crosses national borders to feed his family, the soldier who defends his country or invades another: These are the vivid characters allegedly bringing HIV from Africa, from Haiti, from anywhere but "here."

The possibility of telling the story of AIDS in two ways makes for outrageous retellings that partially secure their credibility through reference to this supposedly factual scientific story. Though scientists would certainly disavow the obvious racism and would most probably point to the inaccuracies in the following (British) National Front account, it nevertheless mobilizes the subtle racism and homophobia on which the scientific account rests. The territorial privilege of the normative and noninfected Western heterosexual white male under siege by deviants—

compressed here into the black bisexual—who exceed their borders puts a face to the vague people who "moved. . . . and travelled":

> THE JEWISH DOMINATED GOVERNMENT AND THE 80 SUBVERSIVE JEWS WHO HAVE INFILTRATED BRITAIN FROM RUSSIA AND EASTERN EUROPE, HAVE (IN ORDER TO DESTROY US), IMPORTED MILLIONS OF BLACKS, THUS BRINGING INTO BRITAIN, AMONG OTHER DISEASES, THE DEADLY KILLER "AIDS." THEY ARE HARDLY LIKE TO EXPOSE THE DEPTH OF THEIR GUILT AND CONSPIRACY BY REVEALING THE FACTS AND EXTENT "AIDS" IS HAVING, ESPECIALLY ON OUR WOMEN FOLK, WHO THROUGH EVIL PROGRAMMING, ARE ENCOURAGED TO ASSOCIATE WITH THE BLACK INVADER.
>
> DR. E. R. FIELDS SAYS "IT HAS NOW BEEN FIRMLY ESTABLISHED THAT THE SPREAD OF 'AIDS' VIRUS TO WHITE FEMALES CAN CLEARLY BE LAID AT THE FEET OF NEGRO BI-SEXUALS AND NEGRO DRUG ADDICTS. THE GROWING TRAGEDY CAN ALSO BE BLAMED ON ALL WHO HAVE PROMOTED THE IDEAS OF 'LIBERAL RACE MIXING.'"
> (*Sic*, British Voice 1988)

In this account, invasion of a once pristine white body politic has been brought about by black people, who are the long arm of another conspiracy: Jews, especially Russian Jews, apparently neither black nor white, intend to use Africans to destroy white womanhood while deceiving the white males who are supposed to protect them ("our women folk"). Unable to actually visualize the individual sexual acts it indicts, the pamphlet lays blame at both the "feet" of the "Negro" and the policies and campaigns that have promoted multiculturalism ("liberal race mixing") as a solution to the social problems faced by immigrants to England from former colonies. Situating Africa as not only the epidemic's starting place (the account also notes that "AIDS SPRANG UP IN AFRICA THROUGH BLACKS HAVING SEX WITH MONKEYS AND THE FACT THAT THE AFRICAN MALES ARE ACCUSTOMED TO HAVING SEX WITH EACH OTHER") but as the place of its densest incidence "THE DISEASE IS RAMPANT ON A MASSIVE SCALE THROUGHOUT BLACK AFRICA"), the account is different from the standard scientific one primarily in tone. Like the scientific version, this popular version slides between place and time, in defiance of all surveillance data, to construct Africa and not the United States as the *place* where the epidemic originated. How did the epidemiologic narrative come to have tropical logics installed so strongly at its core?

Queer Peregrinations

The epidemiologic enterprise is triggered by an increase in the number of cases of a known or unknown medical disorder. Such increases are presumed to result from a change in the biological properties of the pathogens or of the hosts, from a change in the interactions among disease pools, or from some combination of these factors. For example, some bacterial infections are on the rise because the agents have evolved strains resistant to current treatments. Recent increases in epidemic childhood diseases once thought vanquished in the United States appear to have resulted from a decrease in child vaccinations; these hosts are now susceptible to ailments that their older siblings have been vaccinated against. Finally, colds spread from elementary-school classrooms to corporate boardrooms via executives with children; two pools interact because there is a new vector between them. Each of these kinds of change is a feature of the official story that explains AIDS; however, the initial recognition of the syndrome was substantially influenced by a more subtle, rarely considered trigger: a change in health professionals' attitudes about gay men's *health*, that is, by a change in the social construction of what health *is*.

By 1981, when the new medical syndrome was identified, the three-decades-old gay civil rights movement[4] had successfully asserted that gay people formed a civil entity—a minority—and had won increased tolerance for homosexuality from the mental and medical health care establishments. In 1978, the American Psychiatric Association removed homosexuality from its list of psychological disorders (though it retained the subtler category of "ego-dystonic" sexuality—but what queer would not feel a little out of synch in family-values America?). Health care providers were sensitized to the fundamental normalcy— but also to the special needs—of their gay clients. At least in large urban gay ghettos, openly gay people could come to the attention of openly gay or gay-sympathetic health care professionals. That gay men were now considered fundamentally healthy was critical not only in the initial identification of the epidemic but in setting the *terms* of subsequent discourse on HIV and AIDS.

By the late 1970s, these providers were aware that gay men were among the subgroups who experienced sexually transmitted diseases (STDs), and they understood that many gay men avoided treatment out of fear that their sexuality would be revealed to hostile employers, landlords, or family members. Researchers developing the synthetic hepatitis B vaccine had aggressively recruited gay men as medical subjects, even promoting them as heroes who were willing to continue exposing themselves to the virus in hopes that the vaccine would prove effective. To my knowledge, this was the first time that an experimental vaccine for an incurable disease had been tried out under conditions in which people might just as easily have simply changed their behaviors. (I suppose we could include trials of various sorts of contraceptive medications and techniques; pregnancy, in many quarters, is considered as irreversible as viral infection.) Many gay-health educators actually viewed STD-reducing behavior change as an easy task. In the late 1970s, before anyone had even imagined AIDS, some gay periodicals were already promoting condom use, and in San Francisco, there existed at least one group designed to help chronic carriers of hepatitis B meet one another in order to contain their infection among themselves. These preliminary community changes, designed to halt hepatitis B, rest on a political argument drawn from the women's health movement: The historic lack of STD care and especially the denial of information about prevention for gay men were caused by a homophobic medical system. In this late 1970s analysis by gay-health activists, STDs were not a fact of promiscuity but a means through which the state controlled sexuality.

Health activism and related community organizing among gay men constructed a community and provided a potentially radical concept of gay men's special health needs. The appearance of the new disease complex was guaranteed to produce further collective resistance by gay men and their lesbian allies to perceived discrimination. But the early understanding of the new disease complex also guaranteed the adoption of a particular concept of vectors that would survive all political and scientific challenge. Lesbian and gay demands for visibility, a form of political resistance that enabled gay men to respond collectively and rapidly to the epidemic, was easily reversible into the lens of epidemiologic surveillance: The scientific idea of vectors was nestled into the political idea of community. Gay men could be understood as transmission vectors safely trapped within the protective perimeter of "community," a sharply defined "risk group" because their "risk factor" was thought to be coextensive with and exclusive to their group. Although some scientists, in the early 1980s, suggested that gay men's bodies had become altered hosts—broken down out of exhaustion from a fast-lane lifestyle—the bulk of the early epidemiologic and clinical research presumed that the new phenomenon was related to a *new* or newly virulent sexually transmissible agent. This explanation set the science of the 1981–1984 period the task of interrelating the infected bodies through cluster analyses in order to trace the virus's path, characterize its properties, and finally, outrun it with a vaccine. Whereas host-focused, fast-lane theories were criticized as homophobic, agent-focused epidemiology met little political resistance from gay men. The emerging specification of cluster and vector seemed consistent with the new gay civil rights activists' own ideas of community and sexuality.

Epidemiologists described transmission among gay men as multidirectional; HIV circulated freely within the gay community. Unlike women or heterosexual men, gay men were not considered "partners." They were pure vectors limited only by the bounded perimeter of community. Eventually, some women were incorporated into the vectoral scheme; women's bodies were situated between infected man and infectable baby, or they were the shuttle between infected and uninfected men. Like gay men, who when conceptualized as individuals were seen as infectors but when conceptualized as communities were seen as locales of high incidence, prostitutes could also be either vector or place. Indeed, "visiting" a prostitute appears alongside traveling to Africa or Haiti on mid-1980s deferral lists for blood donors.

But for the most part, U.S. discussion of women followed the pattern established in the elaboration of problems of disease/host migration. Nice heterosexual women were safely placed in a home while their men moved about, potentially to the gay spaces that operated as an epicenter and a colony. Under the paternalistic guise of alerting heterosexual women to their potential risk of contracting HIV, popular press writers in the United States almost single-handedly rejected old ideas about male bisexuality to reformulate a new one: "Men [who] may be dangerous to your health" (Norwood 1985, 199). By the mid-1980s, bisexual men were considered to be the true occupants of the closet. If a man-who-had-sex-with-men also had female partners, the media banished him from the gay community. Bisexual men *went to* the dense spaces of homosexuality but did not become "gay." Perilously, he returned, infected with HIV, to the heterosexual home.

Trying out various spatializing tactics, reporters sometimes described the bisexual man as a simple figure of terror who was in the space of his own closet: "a bogeyman . . . cloaked in myth and his own secretiveness" (Nord-heimer 1987, 10). Other writers implicitly compared such men to the new image of the politically and representa-tionally coherent organized gay male community: bisexu-als were "the invisible men . . . without a national organi-zation or sexual agenda" (Heller 1987, 135). Increasingly, though, they were placed in a specific nether region that was opposed to both the subcultural space or ghetto of gay men and the generalized world of straight society; they were men who might "live in towns, cities or suburbs and . . . look and dress like everybody else" while "playing straight with you" (Heller 1987, 135).

But despite women's magazines' differentiation of the gay and the bisexual male, the CDC were satisfied to sim-ply lump gay men and bisexual men into one category based on a single behavior: sex with men. Maybe the me-dia were becoming self-conscious about their own homo-phobia, or maybe the desire to protect women outweighed concerns about the fine line between completely homo-sexual men and bisexual men, but whatever their motive, mainstream media constructed a new kind of pervert. Having to some degree normalized the presence of "nice" gay men—the lawyer next door, the hairdresser, or the florist, with whom the "public" might have only casual contact—the media needed a unique way to describe a kind of man with whom women might actually have sex. Thus, the media did not so much distinguish bisexual men from gay men—no self-respecting straight woman could fail to recognize a queen—as they distinguished them from the truly heterosexual men, whom women would select if they "chose carefully."

Stories like these often began with epidemiology's description of risk groups: homosexual men and the always vague, but female "partners of" heterosexual or bisexual men. But when faced with placing "the man in your life who has a man in his life" (Heller 1987, 134), they switched to the geographic metaphors that characterized tropical conceptions of the disease syndrome. The switch from risk groups to places suggested that the homosexual activity of these frightening men was confined to a specific locale: "Bisexual men and male drug users do have one thing in common, besides their AIDS risk: geography" (Norwood 1985, 199).

Perhaps more subtly, Rabinowitz's "The Secret Sharer: One Woman Confronts Her Homosexual Husband's Death from AIDS" (1990) spatializes the Dr. Jekyll and Mr. Hyde narrative. The now possibly infected wife says, "I married a very different person" (103), and the writer takes pains to distinguish between the husband's localized homosexual life ("In the bathhouses, Alex marched around exhibiting himself" [104]) and his despatialized straight life ("everywhere else, he was the quintessential straight, sometimes homophobic male" [104]). In relation to the "general population," who live in the generalized "everywhere else," homosexuality—and with it, HIV—is proper to, even endemic in, the imagined place of gay community: bathhouses in cities like New York.

Read together, these accounts of disease and its mobility are vertiginous: European and American homosexuals are a "risk group" as long as transmission is considered a "community" issue. But the very places gay men occupy are colonies for their bisexual cohorts, even if gay men are in other accounts *colonists*, especially from the perspective of the governments of developing countries, who, as we shall see below, wished to deny that homosexuality existed within their own borders.

The above-mentioned writers were caught in the contradictions between two ways of telling the story. Although they tried to get the story straight, they quickly abandoned a given logic if it led to conclusions that readers might not want to face: that "straight" men have queer sex and "their" women have straight sex with queer men. Using the tropical model to situate the bisexual male encouraged readers to internalize popular ideas about the fixity of sexual categories rather than to adopt the epidemiologic concept of risk groups. Given that popular media sculpts popular acceptance of health policy, describing bisexual men as transient visitors to the "homosexual" tropics had significant implications. The difference between popular rejection of contact tracing and acceptance of mandatory blood tests for marriage applications showed the extent to which the public, under the influence of such popular media representations as the magazine stories just mentioned, disavowed epidemiologic concepts to align with the narrative strategies of tropical thinking. The epidemiologic rationale for contact tracing did not consider bisexual men to be a special social problem; indeed, the concept of men who have sex with men easily accommodated queers of all sorts in order to advocate safe sex regardless of their self-identity. In epidemiology's ideal world, defined by risk behaviors rather than social labels, both male and female partners of infected persons would be notified and encouraged to be tested for HIV and, regardless of serostatus, to alter their future sexual behavior. (Behavior change was the goal in all early, highly politically contentious tracing programs. Only much later were contact-tracing programs rationalized as a means of getting potentially ill individuals to lifesaving treatments.) In the epidemiologic model, tracking down specific vectors in order to break the chain of transmission would slow the hydra-headed progress of incidence overall.

By contrast, mandatory testing of marriage applicants seemed primarily designed to discover whether men had had sex with other men (and to a lesser degree, whether women had had sex with suspect men and implicitly, whether they had been promiscuous). Unlike contact tracing, which followed the vectoral line anywhere and everywhere, testing of marriage applicants was aimed at discovering whether the male partner had been to the territory occupied by homosexuals (or, more forgivably, that occupied by prostitutes). As the outraged story about "Alex's" double life shows, marriage has no room for sexual deviance of any kind. "Cheating" is a morally reprehensible breech of the marriage contract; a more egregious offense yet is being seropositive, a sign of the crime of making a sham wedding vow. The mandatory test for marriage certificates foreclosed this latter possibility and, especially for the male partner, operated as a passport into state-sanctioned heterosexuality.

This new idea of bisexuality worked well to tropicalize epidemiology's concept of vectors, but it did not fit the local situations and political structures of blame in Third World client states. A second idea of bisexuality emerged as the companion to the U.S. idea of a visitor to an internal colony. The American male bisexual, fixed in his inability to be either gay or straight, spread HIV through his perpetual, diasporal journey between the queer colony and the heterosexual home. Sex tourism presented another option for tropicalizing risk groups in developing countries. Although tourism and sex proved to combine in myriad ways, the most organized versions were early described as a First World prerogative in which men would indulge the sexual desires (especially for homosexual pederasty) that they were too scared to indulge at home. Thus, in representations from and of the Third World, whereas the American queer was mobile, the indigenous male, fundamentally straight, became bisexual for the sake of cash. He was geographically fixed even if he was psychologically labile.

Straight Bodies, Queer Work

The pressure to contain the AIDS epidemic that emerged in the United States and the uncertainty about whether patterns of spread would be roughly the same worldwide sparked an unprecedented official interest in ethnographic studies of sex between men (Abramson and Herdt 1990). Although this work expanded the range of knowledge about same-sex bonds, the underlying agenda of control and the obvious reluctance to let go of comfortable Eurocentric sexual categories resulted in a confusion between "gay men" and same-sex practitioners who go under other names (or no name at all). Part of the problem was that Western ideas about the relationship between AIDS and sexuality arrived in advance of the researchers who hoped to ferret out "indigenous" sexualities. Not only had the media coverage of the epidemic notified the world of a new health phenomenon, but it had also globalized an image of urbanized gay life as the supposed motor of the epidemic. In their urgency to understand diverse forms of homosexuality in order to halt HIV transmission, researchers and research subjects both seemed to have the global media's image in mind. "Other" forms of male-male practice in "other" parts of the world were compared to this ideal case, if only to show that such men did not exist "there." But the untangling of sexual structures was already more complicated than the U.S.–Third World or metropolitan-rural binaries suggested.

Colonial expansion of the nineteenth and twentieth centuries had already mingled forms of same-sex unions that may have, in some earlier time, operated with different symbolic meanings. Although their desirability to practitioners may vary enormously, actual sexual practices are, sadly enough, banally similar. Although sexual practices could not distinguish civilized from uncivilized sex, a combination of racial and class distinctions could figure European and, especially, African sexualities as different from each other. This tautological structure of distinction was recycled in the early debates about why (but never *if*) transmission in Africa was mainly between "heterosexuals." Unlike homosexua*lity* at home, which was thought to result from decadence in the upper classes—*over*civilization—homosexual *practices* found in the colonies were perceived to be *un*civilized. Apparently, Third World queers misread the clues for their organs' "natural" uses, which gender supposedly afforded, or were indifferent to them because they failed to appreciate the role of nuclear heterosexuality as the foundation of civilization. Thus, colonial administrators outlawed many varieties of traditional homosexual marriage or legal partnership that got in the way of tidy management, and Christian missionaries heaped special scorn on homosexual practices (Wekker 1987; Weiringa 1989).

Given the role that routing out homosexualities played in Western constructions of African societies as uncivilized, it was unlikely that *post*colonial governments would acknowledge local homosexualities only a few decades later. Even the trace of these social patterns might again be used to demonstrate a new nation's inferiority. But as long as the specifics of homosexuality were unspeakable, traditionalists found it difficult to prove that the forms disdained by the Europeans were not present. Imagine all the humorous and tragic episodes: People who considered their homosexual practices or relations to be quite ordinary were shocked to discover that it was they themselves about whom the missionaries and magistrates had been speaking when they denounced the vague "crimes against nature." But with the globalization of AIDS, homosexuality got a face and a scientific description. Governments could now very easily show that they had no such homosexuality within their borders or that local forms were an effect of colonialism. Politically savvy postcolonial governments used this anticolonialist version of the tropical thought-style in order to establish that developing countries were essentially heterosexual, while blaming Western homosexuality for bringing any HIV to the tropics. Following this strategy, the left-leaning Panos Institute provides local detail to the ethnographic puzzle of why there might be HIV in Haiti:

> While large numbers of tourists visited briefly from cruise ships, the majority of those who stayed in Haiti were homosexual men, who paid for sex with local men who had wives or girlfriends and considered themselves heterosexual. First the bisexual men become infected, then their female partners, and now Haiti has a full-scale heterosexual AIDS epidemic on its hands. (Panos 1989, 88)

In this troubling nightmare in which the Love Boat has docked on the now-perverted Gilligan's Island, we can almost see the panicked heterosexual tourists mobbing the gangways of the ship from which they have been momentarily ejected by a sinister cruise director. Panos must insist on the brevity of heterosexuals' shore time in order to explain why they could not have infected opposite-sex Haitians for love or money. Apparently, homosexual men have set up some kind of bivouac from which to launch a capitalist invasion that overrides local definitions of sexual identity and the preference for cross-sex practices these are supposed to predict. Queer lucre engenders disease in the tropics because heterosexuality in the colony is premodern; in the face of sparkling dollars, the natives forget what they are. Panos seduces us with an apparently vectoral account—gay men to bisexual men to women—but declines to explain how, given the low probability of female-to-male transmission, this routing could produce the "full-scale heterosexual AIDS epidemic." In order to get the surveillance numbers to balance out, the men who sell sex must also be giving it away to similarly bisexual local men, but that could hardly be characterized as a "heterosexual epidemic."

Most of the HIV-related research on migrants and tourists was conducted long after the idea of the tourist-as-infector had been installed as a central image of a global epidemic (and most such research presented a rather different picture). Western homosexuals, understood to be members of an epidemiologic category when they are at home, suddenly become colonizers when they arrive in a Third World country. The story of their imagined introduction of HIV is narrated as the evil doppelgänger of the story that has justified appealing to tourist dollars in the first place: Only a few people actually engage in serving tourists, but the dollars they obtain trickle out through the rest of the economy. The purely symbolic medium of money is absorbed into an economy that is imagined to otherwise operate through barter and informal exchange. Thus, HIV, like Western money, changes form, shifts from a "homosexual" disease to a "heterosexual" disease. To the extent that tourists are a vector between North and South, HIV transmission is understood to operate in only one direction.

> Haitian researchers have accumulated evidence, through analysis of Haitian blood samples going back over a decade, which they believe shows that the AIDS virus arrived in Haiti with [gay] North American tourists....
>
> The neighboring country of the Dominican Republic, another favoured holiday destination for homosexual men from the United States, has seen a similar shift from homosexual to heterosexual transmission. (Panos 1989, 88)

This tourist version of colonial relations makes the American gay man (a deviant in his homeland) the bearer of disease to the colony; however, the epidemic produced is not among indigenous "homosexuals" but among *het-ero*sexuals. The hurtling queer body goes out of control in the tropics, producing abroad the heterosexual epidemic feared at home. Panos drifts yet further from the practicalities of transmission science when it quotes President Yoweri Museveni of Uganda to even more explicitly link modernization with sexuality: "[AIDS] is the result of European influences—European liberalism, which is good in some respects, has brought a lot of permissiveness, which in a backward society is dangerous" (Panos 1989, 91).

The respective spatializing and temporalizing tendencies of the tropical and epidemiologic thoughtstyles converge here to provide an explanation for how a "backward" society has come into relationship with *both* sides of "European liberalism." In Uganda as an underdeveloped *place*, a place where modernity has arrived *late*, liberalism is an even more frightening epidemic than HIV—or it is at least HIV's fatal cofactor. But in Uganda as the final frontier, a place with no less-modern place to pass its infection *to*, AIDS cannot, finally, be incorporated into the temporal scheme. This kind of moment in telling the story of AIDS is the point of the most dangerous narrative implosion: Whenever a temporal narrative indicates a *last place*, there is a breath, a pause, while HIV *takes root*, becomes *endemic*. In and for that moment, HIV arrives. Vectorality and time are only recovered if and when that place sets a body loose to form a link with a new place. Only then is diasporal movement rewritten as part of an infection chain.

In the early 1980s, this complicated linking of modernity, but especially capitalism, with supposedly new sexualities, but especially practices people would only engage in for money, allowed governments to deny there would be an HIV epidemic in their country. In the second part of the 1980s, they used the very same logic to explain how foreign homosexuals had produced a domestic epidemic among their own heterosexuals. Dancing between two means of making homosexuality Other (a hurtling Western body or something that Westerners misread as queer), few governments ever conceded that there was much transmission among local men who have sex with men.

A classic example of the danger this response represented for local modes of homosexuality occurred when a representative of the South African Ministry of Mines set out to discover what safe-sex education his workers might need. None, he concluded, based on data that suggested that although miners did form homosexual relationships while away from their homes, little anal intercourse was practiced (or acknowledged) (Whiteside 1988; Moody 1988). On the most obvious level, Alan Whiteside's conclusion makes sense: Why educate people who are not practicing unsafe sex? His report might even be considered antihomophobic, protecting these same-sex relationships from the scorn they would surely receive if they were to come to be understood as "gay." His report might even be considered anticolonialist, since safe-sex campaigns lay the queer body open to state scrutiny.[5]

At the time of his study, Whiteside was among the most advanced economic and health planners because he accepted the existence and normative importance of forms of homosexuality that did not look like those in the West, or indeed, did not look like the communities and activities of organized white gay men in his own country. Confounded by the split imposed by Patterns One and Two, safe-sex campaigns in South Africa laid bare the sexual presuppositions that underlay apartheid and colonialism generally: The "white" campaign was concerned with homosexual sex, while the "black" campaign was concerned with the preservation of "the family." Contemporaneous campaigns in adjacent African countries commonly argued that unsafe heterosexual sex destroyed the family (a project already nearly accomplished by colonialism and by ill-conceived postcolonial development schemes). The South African campaigns of the late 1980s were only more blatant in targeting information regarding homosexuality to white men while organizing campaigns concerned with heterosexual sex through representations of black nationals in and as families.

Of course, there are numerous explanations for Whiteside's apparent farsightedness: the economic interests he officially represented, the white racist anxieties he had to negotiate even if he did not endorse them, the homophobic anxiety produced by whites and attributed to (and perhaps also held by) blacks. But actually, when I talked to him briefly, Whiteside seemed like a nice enough guy: sincere, honest, and critical of South African policies. He seemed to be trying to resist, from his important government post, the worst of white racism in order to improve the lot of black miners. Indeed, Whiteside does not need to be a bad guy: The policy frame in which he had to operate and its connection to global AIDS policy meant that whatever he said and did at an international conference were bound to be read through and to reinforce the GPA's pattern structure. Indeed, even Dunbar Moody, the anthropologist on whose research Whiteside relied, cannot escape being reread through the genocidal logic that acknowledges homosexuality as "real" only when its practice results in potential self-extinction. Moody's findings about the diversity of sexual and affective practices among men who understand themselves to be engaged in (and even to prefer) relationships with men fell prey to prescriptions about "sex in the age of AIDS": Whiteside can read differences in practice only as differences in potential rates of HIV transmission. Instead of promoting male miners' sexuality as *models* of safe sex, the minister concluded that the miners were not appropriate subjects for the type of prevention messages that had been aimed at (white) "homosexuals." Even if he accepts that miners at least transiently build same-sex bonds, the minister cannot imagine them as "homosexuals" because they do not engage in "real sex."

Men Who Have Sex with Men

Moody's was the kind of work on sexual relations pursued by constructionist social scientists doing AIDS research. By about 1989, advisers to the GPA were able to use this new science to gain official adoption and normalization of the term "men who have sex with men" (MSM). Although unwieldy, this term represented an important conceptual move away from the European and American tendency to ground homosexuality in psychic processes or to posit queerly desiring bodies as proto-gay subjects who could be organized into an identity and a community. The tension between the globalized image of gay men and the local men who have sex with men did not so much smash stereotypes as create a domain in which both internationalist and transnationalist ideas of queerness could be used to advantage. The MSM rubric made it possible for GPA's HIV educators to work closely and sensitively with local homosexualities. In turn, individuals from such locales offered local details about their complex sexuality, which lent credence to the social constructionist theories and showed the utility of the new MSM designation. The visibility and contacts local queers achieved by entering HIV-prevention work and, critically, by increasing their participation in the international lesbian and gay movement helped convince health ministers that their citizens already practiced "native" forms of homosexuality. This visibility both consolidated the gay movement's internationality and reinforced the cultural differences within—and finally the incoherence of—the category "gay." For individuals, participating in global AIDS politics meant producing themselves as "gay" in order to insist on the specificity of their "original" homosexuality, and thus, the lack of universality of the American gay ideal.

Unfortunately, these real-life struggles over essentialist and social-constructionist uses of sexual nomenclatures could not overcome the tendency in safe-sex discourse itself to insist on a fixed link between sexual identity and practices of pleasure. After all, the growing acceptance of global homosexualities—at least in the abstract—was substantially a result of desires to change sexual behavior. Instead of calling attention to practices that needed modification, the avowal and disavowal of identities increased the possibilities for ignoring safe-sex advice. Educators assumed that there was a core of basic words that everyone would understand as referring to a fixed set of acts. Readers of educational pamphlets were expected to sort out for themselves the local terms related to myriad identities; they were required to translate advice that was stripped of cultural marks and that used the driest descriptors of sexual acts. By presuming readers would overlay their particular identities onto supposedly neutrally described practices, educators overlooked the ways in which particular relations between practices and identities result in strong attachments to the ideography of practices that had produced differing identities in the first place.

The activists' insight that risk is not who one is but what one does turned out not to be exactly equal to the educators' distinction between identity and practice. Identity is not so much the recognition that one is what one does, but rather the recognition that one is the sort of person who recognizes the value of an act like that. In trying to break the link between particular Western connotations of, say, anal sex as they arose within discussions of AIDS, educators hoped to make it possible for individuals who engaged in this practice under some other symbolic regime to recognize that "safe sex" applied to them, even if they did not hold—or even if they actively refused—a similar identity. Unfortunately, to the extent that the value of an act is embedded in a social world that understands itself through the shorthand "gay," to talk only of practice appears to "de-gay" even anal sex between men. The tactic of stripping the referent of its most powerful signs proved impossible. The result was a safe-sex Esperanto that was comprehensible to everyone but meaningful to no one.

This complex construction and disavowal of identity in the Third World (and in the endotropics of the developed world, that is, the black and gay ghettos) produced a fatal spiral for prevention activism. When safe-sex discourse tried to persuade appropriate (if "closeted") subjects to convert to condom use, it collaborated in constructing intercourse as both the sine qua non and principal danger of sex. Perpetually vilifying intercourse in order to dissuade its practice narrowed the images of safe sex. Safe-sex advice perpetually invoked unsafe sex, without reminding men that most of what they already did was safe. Reducing safe sex to the symbol of the condom tended, even in the most savvy projects, to accidentally produce Westernized, urbanized sexual subjects among men who have sex with men under other symbolic regimes.

As the Moody work showed, when researchers did locate MSM, they discovered that in fact MSM do not, or do only under some circumstances, engage in anal intercourse with other men. They *already* practice safe sex, but not as such. Educators believed that in order to sustain these already safe cultural norms, Westernized notions of unsafe sex had to be introduced. This was difficult to do in a colonial context without suggesting that intercourse, the now-distinguishing preoccupation of urban Western gay discourse, is the "real" form of homosexuality. Paradoxically, Western safe-sex programs directed toward men who have sex with men tried to introduce intercourse in order to discourage its practice.

The production and naturalization of homosexuality was even more obviously problematic when men from differing sexual cultures met on a socioscape, now partially framed through globalized concepts of safe sex. For example, one study conducted in the context of the HIV epidemic suggests that male Mexican migrant workers adopted new sexual practices while in southern California, including male-male sex and oral and anal intercourse (Bronfman and Minello 1992, D423). Although migrants denied continuing male-male sexual relations upon their return to Mexico, both anal and oral sex were incorporated into their sexual repertoires with both casual and regular female partners. The interviews also suggest that the men's recognition of the stigma in Mexico of the behaviors they engaged in while migrating made it more difficult for them to adopt safer techniques generally. The men were highly informed about HIV transmission and its interruption, but because of the complex bicultural segmentation of their sexual relationships at home and in migration settings, the men were disinclined to identify themselves as engaging in risk behaviors or to adopt risk-reducing practices. Like bisexuality practiced in a single locale, personal risk seemed to be assessed from the standpoint of the "safe identity"; that is, rather than thinking of themselves as men who had sex with men, and therefore the subjects of safe-sex advice, these men seemed to think of themselves as heterosexuals and therefore "safe."

The extent to which migrant workers form relationships with men who are part of more openly gay communities is unknown. Although homosexual relationships formed while away may be similar in form and effect to relationships with "town wives," with whom the same men may also have relations, the power relations between men are significantly different than those between men and women, and the power relations between men who do and those who do not wish to disclose their homosexuality also differs. As several studies of Anglo-European tourism in developing countries have suggested, the person perceived to be more culturally powerful may also be perceived to be responsible for initiating and sustaining safer-sex practices. To migrating men who have homosexual relations in the host country, it may seem that local residents are the experts on the need for safe sex, while the Anglo-European gay men to whom they look for advice are used to operating in an environment of sexual negotiation between approximate equals.

The terminological shifts from "homosexual" to "gay" to "men who have sex with men" track sophisticated changes in concepts about male sexuality: from gender of object of affection to social identity to specificity of practice. Like efforts to find the least culturally overdetermined words to describe safe sex, the adoption of "men who have sex with men" sanitized sex and minimized the probable social differences among homosexual actors. Although it seemed that more homosexual subcultures and modes of practice had come to light, there was a hidden paradox in the new global discourse of sexuality. Obscured were the existing subtle, but very real, costs of living a life outside any local cultural norm. Like the explicitly colonialist and missionary antiperversion drives of an earlier era, safe-sex campaigns—though inadvertently—seemed to construct a particular notion of heterosexuality as the norm against which MSM were to be calculated as alternate or different. But heterosexualities were also more complex than global AIDS discourse suggested.

Heterosexuality for Hire

Since the nineteenth century, public health officials have believed that prostitutes were central conduits for and sentinels of disease. Prostitutes' dual position in health policing—as perpetrators and as messengers—only reinforced fears of longer standing that, unleashed, women's sexuality would engulf humanity. Even in the abstract, prostitution was thought to be symptomatic of a society's decline. This compound fear of and interest in women's role in sexual commerce was reinvigorated when early cases of AIDS were identified in the United States among women believed to be prostitutes. Prostitutes' rights activists quickly got involved, and many longtime activists from around the world were involved in the GPA's prostitute project during the Mann years. Prostitutes around the world were already organizing against harassment and for improved access to health care. Thus, the GPA was for a time a center of a variety of different approaches to prostitution: empowering women, getting prostitutes out of sex work, and treating them as a public health problem.

The Eighth International Conference on AIDS (1992) hosted a three-day symposium on "prostitution"; a central aspect of the symposium concerned language. Many of the women who engage in acts that epidemiologists count as prostitution, but especially feminists who have understood prostitution through a broad antipatriarchal analysis, preferred the term "sex work," which emphasizes labor issues, to the term "prostitution," which seems to carry a hopeless array of negative images and meanings. However, for some women, keeping the term "prostitute" reclaimed a disdained identity and recalled a history of oppression of women's sexuality that the term "sex work" dehistoricized. Yet others pointed out that whatever complex of colonialist ideas "prostitution" encapsulated, the term "sex work" was even more subtly and problematically Eurocentric. Rooted in a Marxist feminism that attempts to shift debates about bartered sex away from issues of morality and onto issues of labor, the term "sex work," at least as used in global HIV policy debates, promoted capitalist concepts of market and economy. Organizing women as sex workers attempted to construct a notion of identity—as a worker—for women engaging in a wide variety of erotic performances. Grouping these disparate kinds of activity under the rubric "sex work" seemed to repeat a confusion that had earlier arisen in safe-sex education efforts: the effort to promote safe sex among homosexual men by producing identification with a gay community, which required the introduction of a thoroughly Western idea of individual identity.

In the case of so-called sex work, in order for domestic barters, including sex, to make sense as *work*, safe-sex educators had to insist on a separation between private (the properly constructed home) and public domains of labor, the very distinction that is criticized by Western feminists ("the personal is political"). But in many of the cultures coping with the epidemic, this political and economic separation was not salient, or if partially accomplished, it was linked with postcolonial development plans to which local people were already hostile. Like the obsessive reminders of the danger of anal intercourse that seemed necessary to the then-current logic of safe sex, insistence on the term "sex work" required the introduction of the very framework for sexuality that activists hoped to overcome: Sex must be *privatized* in order to make it public as formal work. This strategy could not finally escape the moralism that some feminists argued the term "prostitute" entailed. In the absence of an established professional social role to reconstruct, that is, the role of prostitute, the concept of sex work makes paid-for sex appear to be a commodified substitute for what properly happens at home.

Although they are crucial to women's survival, local and global discourses about sex work collide in particularly hazardous ways. Throughout the world, women systematically trade companionship and sex in order to supplement their cash, and the names and meanings for these practices vary enormously. But from the perspective of researchers working from the epidemiological thought-style, these situations are all lumped together as prostitution, a particular form of heterosexuality characterized by higher than average sexual partner change for women, accompanied by explicit economic exchange. But this categorical scheme, whatever similarities in transmission demographics can be shown across sociocultural and geopolitical spaces, misses the fact that social differences among forms of sexual barter strongly affect the extent to which women can effect safe sex.

It is easy to see that the willingness to practice safe sex, and even the perception of the need for it, will differ across both locales and types of relationship. For example, in many parts of the world (including most U.S. suburbs), these bargains are simply understood as "going out," a means of supplementing a single woman's meager resources, perhaps only by offering sex in exchange for a nice dinner and a movie. But in the same city, and in a very particular way in postcolonial countries with extensive experience with Europeans, there is *also* a concept of prostitution. This exchange, although a financial analogue to "going out," is understood as devoting one's attention to selling sex and favors to a particular clientele, perhaps *European men*.

Colonial governance and other changes in local economies have regularly altered patterns of sexual barter, but the history of local and local-translocal sexual formations has not been widely studied. The direction of change is probably variable. For example, European styles of prostitution were probably superimposed on existing types of transaction, some of which may have become less appealing to some women. Imagine the first case: He wants to pay for sex and leave? You mean I don't have to wash his clothes and cook his food? Here, prostitution becomes a profession rather than a supplementary avocation, a social role with a deeply ambivalent relation to colonial ideas about sexuality. Insofar as some women elected to fill this job, a *new* pattern of sexual barter must have emerged, one overtly linked to European men and their sexual ideologies. Presumably, the old and new patterns of sexual barter continue to have different symbolic meanings, and women who engage in them organize their lives in different ways. Women who "go out" may actively reject the idea that they are "prostitutes," viewing that form of sex trade as immoral or as "modern" and in violation of their traditional gender roles. "Going out" is different from sex with a domestic partner and different again from prostitution. "Going out" may simply conform to normative expectations; it may simply be an unthought dimension of urban working women's identity as feminine persons. By contrast, "prostitution" in the same place would require another form of identity, perhaps one linked with participation in a Europeanized sociosexual order.

These speculative differences in identity that varying forms of sexual exchange entail mean not only that researchers misunderstand the objects of their study, but also that the "targets" of education programs may not see themselves as the women to whom advice about safe sex is directed. Differences in self-conception and gender-role identity are critical. If, for example, condoms are heavily associated with prostitution, then women who "go out" may not perceive their utility or may be actively hostile toward their use.

The ready availability of media that promulgated a cluster of generalized but universal stereotypes about AIDS and its subjects exacerbated local differences. One strikingly incorrect idea that was suggested was that any woman who had AIDS was a prostitute. Worse yet, because prostitutes' rights organizing had already largely focused on women, another conflation occurred in the global discourse about

AIDS and sex work: Sex workers were largely presumed to be women, and women at risk were assumed to be prostitutes.[6] On the other hand, men who sell sex to men were lumped together as men who have sex with men, a division repeated in the risk-group-oriented project divisions of the GPA. This gender asymmetry duplicated the active-passive split that is supposed to characterize male versus female sexuality. This conceptualization, I will show below, also underlies the pattern scheme used by GPA. Whereas men sell bodies that are theirs to dispose of, women sell bodies that more properly belong to men, their families, or society as a whole. This gender difference in the construction of the sex trade was politically problematic, because it cast prostitutes as the object of policing not to protect her but to protect men, children, family, and society. On the scientific level, it resulted in fatal misinterpretations of epidemiologic data regarding who (predominantly men or women) were the usual clientele of male versus female sex workers.

In fact, for the first decade of the epidemic, most policy about prostitution was developed from cultural stereotypes and generalized impressions about the workers themselves. Almost no research was conducted on the clients of sex workers, in part because (male) researchers did not want to violate clients' privacy (though they were happy enough to violate the privacy of sex workers, who are at much greater risk of arrest) and in part because customers were thought to be difficult to contact. It may be true that few men acquired a social identity as "john" in the way that workers were assumed to acquire the identity "prostitute." At least in Anglo-European countries, hiring sex workers was viewed simply as a male prerogative, not as a source of oppositional identity, that is, an identity that made a man a participant in an antiestablishment subculture and a potential activist against laws or social mores that discriminated against prostitutes and johns (Zalduondo 1991, 232–33). In addition, the fact that johns had exercised this male privilege was taken as evidence of their sexual activity, of their ineluctible heterosexuality. But this culturally bound linkage of heterosexuality with action and commerce proved to be a mistake of dramatic proportions that epidemiologists have still not accepted, despite research that demonstrates the degree to which male prostitutes have female partners and johns have male partners.

When researchers finally began to study clients, they were in for a big surprise. Two studies, conducted in Atlanta, Georgia, and in London, shattered social stereotypes about the presumed "heterosexuality" of male clients who hire women for sex. The London study (Day 1992) showed that 37 percent of johns interviewed reported past sexual contact with men, with condom use highest in their commercial contacts. The Atlanta study (Elifson, Boles, and Doll 1992) compared the ten-year sexual histories of clients of male sex workers to those of female sex workers' clients. Men who had initially been identified as clients of male sex workers had twice the rate of HIV seroprevalence (37 percent) as those who had initially been identified as clients of female sex workers (17 percent). However, among the clients of male sex workers, 64 percent had had sex with both men and women, and among the clients of female sex workers, 43 percent had had sex with both men and women. In addition, 39 percent of clients of male sex workers had also hired female sex workers, and 29 percent of clients of female sex workers had also hired male sex workers.

These two studies demonstrated that paid or unpaid risk-relevant homosexual activity among prostitutes' clients is not only not exclusive to "gay" clients, but may also constitute a significant but poorly described route of HIV transmission *to* female sex workers, who had been presumed to contract HIV from needle sharing or from heterosexual sex with needle users. These findings raised serious questions about two assumptions that were fundamental to HIV epidemiology *and to the definition of Pattern Two ("heterosexual" predominance) in the GPA scheme:* first, that clients of male and of female sex workers are distinct populations, and second, that in transactions between (non-drug-injecting) male clients and female sex workers, he was more at risk from her than she was from him. These studies, which were among the first to analyze clients as potentially infectious rather than as *at risk from* sex with prostitutes, show what prostitute organizers had long insisted: At least in regard to HIV, sex workers needed to use condoms to protect themselves, not their clients. In addition, condom campaigns, which had focused primarily on heterosexual or on gay and bisexual men, had to reconsider the range of practices of the men they were trying to reach. Engaging in sex that was perceived to be "commercial" might enable men who were otherwise mainly homosexual to sustain a heterosexual self-identification in the face of a lifetime practice associated with gay identity. Educators tended to think of this as "closeted" or "repressed," but the masculinity-conveying power of buying sex may mean that clients really do experience themselves as Other to the men whose immediate services, or even longer-term gender-role structured relationships, they buy.

Like gay men in the United States, prostitutes around the world were constructed as a tropic. Whether or not they actually worked in a specific locale, they were understood as the immutable place of heterosexual commerce; clients were constructed only as transient visitors. In fact, most large-scale epidemiologic studies looked at STD/HIV rates among sex workers generally, not at rates among specific sex workers over time. Researchers did quickly realize that because of police sweeps and professional turnover, a large number of the women studied at any given time were absent from the next sample, taken at a later time. By 1990, critics of global policy argued that both the pattern scheme and the notions of geographical safety that epidemiologists were trying to contest were shot through with racist and sexist stereotypes. Concern about Asia, finally an area of focus for the complicated bifocal lens of global policy and global resource allocation, threatened to undo the official narrative schemes. The Asian epidemic was thought to have proliferated through the sale of sex, but from Westerners' perspective, women were finally cast as the victims, both of foreign men and of their own governments, who policed them as deviants in their own locales. Suddenly, the entire Western policy enterprise was concerned with the oppression of women! But gendered concepts—even the apparently neutral epidemiologic notion of time—overdetermined the direction of HIV education and policy once the "late-blooming" epidemic in Asia began to decimate women.

Feminizing "Asian AIDS"

It is fairly obvious that stereotypes about sexuality complicated the pattern designations used by the GPA. AIDS was initially linked with homosexual practice, but even the emergence of substantial numbers of AIDS cases among heterosexuals did not diminish the association of AIDS with sexual deviancy. Instead, heterosexuals who happened to contract HIV were assumed to be practicing some bizarre form of sex. Because their route of transmission was believed to be from prostitutes,[7] the men diagnosed with HIV in Africa were counted as heterosexual by Western researchers, with their ethnocentric, even voyeuristic definitions. The misunderstandings about Western clients' sexuality were projected onto Africans, which reinforced the idea that the clients of prostitutes are, de facto, heterosexual. This "discovery" of "heterosexual AIDS" in about 1984 only made it easier for the U.S. media and the scientists themselves to believe that only perverse bodies were subject to HIV, for African heterosexuality was persistently described as perverse, precultural, and primitive.[8]

Ironically, the initial *lack* of reported cases of AIDS in Asia through the 1980s contributed to the association of HIV with another kind of sexual perversion. Although cases of HIV and AIDS were described among Asians in the early to middle 1980s, HIV only became visible as a problem *for* Asia when it appeared among sex workers, transforming sex workers from a sexual/tropical home away from home for Westerners into a vector within Asia. Because Asian sexuality was stereotyped as passive, as primarily capable of receiving but not passing on HIV, early low incidence figures were interpreted within the tropical framework as a reflection of a kind of immunity rather than as an artifact of HIV's late arrival, as the epidemiologic model would hold. But by 1992, at the Eighth International Conference on AIDS in Amsterdam, HIV was represented as now having become endemic to Asia and as being passed among members of the Asian migrant groups and underclasses. Once "Asian AIDS" was launched, blame concerning the diasporal relations of migrant Western homosexuals was subordinated to hysteria about heterosexual vectoral transmission. "Asian AIDS" was likened to "African AIDS," not to the unmarked but unmistakably queer AIDS of Anglo-America.

Researchers and policy makers interpreted the low relative incidence of HIV in Asia and among nongay Asian Americans as an indicator of sexual conservatism, even asexuality, on the part of Asians. Many of the first AIDS cases diagnosed in Asia occurred among hemophiliac men or were attributed to male-male sex between locals and traveling Western homosexuals. Chun-Jean Lee, the director-general of the Department of Health of the Taiwan Provincial Government, tried to negotiate the different implications of the epidemiologic and tropical narratives in his description of the trajectory of HIV as it made its way to his tiny country:

> AIDS has been identified only within the past ten years in central Africa; from there it quickly spread to Haiti and then to the U.S. and to Europe. It came very late to

Taiwan: in December 1984 an American transiting Taiwan was found to have full-blown AIDS. This triggered our first major concern over the fatal disease. However a rapid increase in the number of AIDS patients locally, the spread of the disease to other parts of Taiwan, development of AIDS among HIV carriers in hemophiliacs, the diversification of risk groups—all have followed the same pattern seen in Western countries and throughout the world. (Lee, C.-J., 1989, xii)

Two crucial elements in this otherwise stock account leave open Taiwan's future options for retelling the story of AIDS: the relativity of time and the exceptionality of Africa (and heterosexual transmission). First, though the period for viewing the epidemic is said to be short—"ten years"—the American transiting in 1984 is described as arriving "very late," invoking the GPA's nomenclature to suggest that an Asian epidemic could still be prevented, but only if homosexuals and faulty blood products were prevented from entering there.

It is, of course, a simple fact that at a time when the Western countries were overwhelmed by case numbers, Asia's HIV count was low. But epidemiology and tropical medicine interpret this in different ways, ways that have enormously different implications for how a country should respond. Early incidence could only be considered low *in comparison to the realization in the West of how high numbers could go.* New York once had low numbers, as did Boston, Pittsburgh, Wichita, Dubuque, and Tiny Town, USA. At least in retrospect, early incidence in *any* epidemic will always seem low; it is part of the *definition* of epidemic that the numbers are suddenly relatively high. But the crucial difference in this account lies in how the conditions for local spread are perceived. Instead of viewing Asians as a series of potentially connected bodies in which the chain of a future series of transmissions could be interrupted, tropical logic kicked in to conceive of Asia as a place in which HIV could not spread.

Second, when the director-general relies on the now-standard account to explicitly situate Africa as the epidemic's origin, he can insist that "Western countries" are the epicenters relevant to Asia; that is, West-East movement is his paradigm for dispersion in Taiwan. If he can deny the possibility of significant levels of transmission between local homosexuals, he can deny that Taiwan will see many "Taiwanese" cases. But this attempt to refigure Taiwan, and Asia more generally, as more-like-America was neither adopted by the U.S. researchers nor accepted by the GPA, which sustained the idea of Asian difference. Though African and Asian AIDS were labeled Patterns Two and Three, by the 1980s, the African and Asian cases had come to represent two extremes in Western images of the epidemic, two different visions of the West's epidemiologic future. Each pattern held out a lesson: If you don't use condoms, you'll turn into Africa; if you don't have sex, you can be Asia. Africa is always infectious, Asia is always infectable, and a white body is precariously suspended between them. Invoking and displacing the obvious gender constructions encapsulated in the pattern scheme—and the scheme's failure to escape the cultural stereotypes that accrue to regions—epidemiologists seemed uninterested in how African men became infected, how women within Asia might become infected, and why homosexuals everywhere continued to become infected despite massive safe-sex campaigns.

Interestingly, by equating Taiwan's epidemic with that in the West, the director-general must tacitly accept the presence of native homosexuals. His colleagues cope with the problems such an admission might entail by arguing away the possibility of rampant transmission between men. One study of Taiwan's local homosexual men provided considerable detail about the now-admitted but taboo native homosexuality; apparently *Taiwanese* homosexuals do not engage in the dangerous practices that have spread HIV among their equivalents in the licentious West!

> According to the statements on the questionnaires, kissing was the most common sexual practice but, after extensive interviewing, male homosexuals often admitted anal intercourse as well.... None described practices of "fisting."... Low prevalence of HIV-1 was detected in several high risk groups. If the results of the questionnaire and interview are accepted as reliable, homosexual behavior in Taiwan appears to be much less promiscuous than in the western world. (Lee, H.-C., et al. 1989, 65)

Taiwan's homosexuals are apparently constitutionally passive, barely sexual at all. By extension, Asian resistance to the epidemic is primordial, a vague, almost feminine incapacity to become infected except by outsiders. By any temporal logic—in fact, by the very logic that concluded that intervention in Africa was "too late"—Asia, as the place where AIDS "arrived late," should have been an ideal candidate for aggressive prevention campaigns. Sadly, risk-reduction programs truly arrived late, and the tropical logic was used to justify the failure to act.

Sex Tourism

The first Western discussions about HIV in Asia came through "exposés" of Australian and U.S. sex tourism. This collision between Orientalism and Victorian sexual attitudes produced a frenzy of pseudoconcern for Asian women and children, who were supposedly being swept away by imported Western perversions. These articles were largely prompted by moral panic over the range and dispersion of sexual differences rather than by serious consideration of Westerners' cultural responsibility. Under the guise of protecting supposedly helpless women, children, and nonperverse men, Western governments and media pundits now had another rationale for policing their own deviant populations. But the reports on sex tourism also reinforced Western figurations of Asians as drugged sexual deviants: women and children so exotic they lured Western men to their beds, Asian men too drugged to care. Indeed, sex tourists (in fact, many are themselves Asians on business trips or true sex tourists—men traveling specifically for sex—going from wealthier to poorer countries) were described as seeking sexual outlets for practices stigmatized at home. Homosexual sex tourists, who were presumed to be both closeted at home and unconcerned about their partners abroad, were cast as extremely likely to spread HIV abroad. This complex of media representations and the tropical idea of AIDS on which they relied doubly feminized Asia in the context of global AIDS policy: Asia was passive ("AIDS *arrives* late") and, like the popular Anglo trope of the prematurely developed pubescent girl, Asia was alluring beyond her own comprehension, *attracting* fatal attention.

The transnational sex trade may well be a factor in the health-planning equation. Abuse of poor—most often female—participants is and should be of concern to human rights and workers' rights advocates, but not because sex tourism is the final manifestation of what Frantz Fanon half a century ago dubbed "a dying colonialism." The West's admission to its role in *this* form of colonial intercourse is a cover for its participation in much more sophisticated, covert forms it has no intention of giving up. Emphasizing this complex victimization of women and children whom the West has abandoned in every other possible way is appealing because sexuality is the one domain of global regulation in which the West still feels confident of its moral correctness. By explicitly blaming perversion on itself, or rather, on some of its least-respected members, the West can go through the motions of making up for its colonial misuse of foreign people and their lands. By treating Asia largely as the object of tourists' fantasies and focusing on the active culpability of individual sex tourists, the West can play out its own fantasy of rescuing the damsel in distress. Western health officials thereby avoid acknowledging that their neglect of Asian countries is partly responsible for the late development of HIV-prevention programs in Asian locales.

Planners failed to examine the sociopolitical conditions of local sex-tourism sites, ultimately conflating people who traveled to find sex with those who happened to have sex while away from home. The most visible result of concern about sex on the road was a spate of advice for travelers and tourists, in which policy makers attempted to cope with sexuality's labile possibilities:

Sex Tourism

For both visitors and the host country, tourism becomes a risky business when tours and sex are sold together. In some cases, as in Thailand, a country's tourist industry is heavily based on the packaged sex holiday, catering for those who go abroad to do things they would probably never do at home. (Sabatier 1988, 88)

Q: How can the sexual spread of AIDS be prevented while traveling?

Do not have sex with prostitutes (male or female) or casual acquaintances, even in countries claiming that they have no AIDS problem.... If having sex with someone who may be infected, men should use a condom each time from start to finish, and women should make sure that their partner uses one.... Finally, remember that the fewer sexual partners you have, the lower your risk of exposure to the virus that causes AIDS. (WHO 1989a, 35)

In their confusion about who might infect whom and about *where* AIDS might be, these two bits of advice about travel and HIV ignore the problem of getting *anyone* to actually practice safe sex, a problem most educators agree stems from the complex interaction between personal identities and social power. Both the Panos Institute and the WHO assume that individuals participate in personal power relations in the same way that their countries participate on the global stage. Especially in the Panos text, this collapse of individual possibilities with national destiny suggests that power operates only on the axis of master to client state, with the sex tour destinations living out an especially odious kind of dependency. But even in the WHO advice, destination countries are described as "claiming that they have no AIDS problem." It is easy to see that this more innocuous-seeming advice also imagines a master state–client state relationship between the partners to this sex. Given that both Pattern One and Pattern Two countries are said to have massive cases of AIDS, only a Pattern Three country could even try to claim they had "no AIDS problem." These explicit and oblique invocations of postcolonial cultural dynamics suggest that there is only one axis of power difference: Travelers carry with them the power of master countries and impose upon client countries and their hapless residents. This ignores power differences that accrue from gender, sexuality, class, or culture. For example, Western women—who most would argue have less power in sexual relationships with Western men—are presumed, by virtue of being Western, to have more power than those they find in the client-state setting. Reciprocally, the above conflation of national and sexual power misreads the degree of social agency of male sex workers, who, although potentially disempowered in relationship to monied male sex tourists, still have greater power than their local female partners. These gradients of power difference are multiple and complex, as research on sex and travel began to suggest. For example, for the first decade of the epidemic, Third World purveyors of sex were presumed uniquely incapable of demanding safe sex, and sex tourists were presumed uniquely capable of refusing it. However, studies of tourists suggest that Western women travelers are no more successful at gaining compliance to safe sex abroad than at home, and studies of male sex workers do not suggest that they engage in safer practices with their local partners. As I suggested above, studies do suggest that Third World participants often look to their Western partners for cues about practicing safe sex, and it is not at all clear that the Westerners (especially gay men) do not welcome and encourage the practice safe sex.

In the first advice quoted above, the attempt to hold more powerful *nations* responsible for the transformation of colonial relations into tourist relations leads the avowedly critical Panos Institute to fail to recognize that transnational sexual relations are operating more against the state than under its watchful eye. As the Panos Institute frames it, the only solution to the problem is for an extranational body to step in and protect developing countries afflicted with sex tourism. But this policing would finally have to have an object, and the conflation of nation and individual would certainly revert to its individual form: The bodies of the only barely disguised Western perverts who "do things they would probably never do at home." As individual advice, this is vague at best. As a policy logic, it denies that the providers of sexual services might have elaborate patterns of desire and practice independent of the sex tourists whom they serve.

In the second case, the traveling body needs to protect itself from the unquestioned duplicity of countries that, like the proverbial lover, lie about their infection. These two international policy organizations' incapacity to decide where AIDS *is* (in bodies or in places?) and how it *moves* (vectorally from the First World or in the bodies returning to it?) is not coincidental. We can see in relief here that the neat stories we tell about AIDS, drawing as they do on slightly different but related medical thought-styles, implode to construct and reconstruct bodies, places, and movement in irregular and unpredictable ways. This realization sheds a different light on the sudden burst of interest in those places where AIDS "arrived late."

It is suspicious that the concern (circa 1992) about HIV in Asia and especially in Thailand occurred at the same moment that scientists announced their interest in conducting vaccine trials there. In 1990, I predicted that the ways in which Africa was described—Africans won't use condoms; Africa is a disaster; in Africa, AIDS is a disease of poverty (rather than of individual acts)—would be used to justify the conduct there of HIV vaccine trials that would not pass ethical muster elsewhere. I was only partly correct: Some of that vaccine research continues, but by the early 1990s, the temporal logic that had once promoted Africa as the original locale of "AIDS" had begun to be used to suggest that Africa was already lost. Research attention was therefore refocused on more-cooperative lands that science might possibly save. Thus, by the mid-1990s, Asia, "where AIDS arrived late," met the ideological conditions necessary to conduct the highly controversial HIV vaccine trials.[9] The poignant rallying cry of gay communities of the late 1980s—that education is the only vaccine—had backfired. If scientists could convince society that education cannot work, then vaccine trials, whatever their ethical status, were, ipso facto, the only hope. They became a humanitarian effort to avert an imminent disaster rather than an ethical disaster that refuses to improve and support lifesaving social and behavioral change.

The media coverage of sex tourism proved crucial to this ideologically based campaign for vaccine trials. Writers insisted that uncontrollable elements propelled the Asian sex trade. Both male sex drive and the culture of poverty were said to drive men and women to sell themselves. In the face of these powerful natural (or naturalized, in the case of brute colonial existence) forces, safe-sex campaigns were said to be unworkable, and placebo-controlled vaccine trials—which require continued transmission if any results are to be achieved—would therefore be ethical. "Saving Asia" became the final chapter in the larger temporal narrative proposed by epidemiology, justifying the very stereotypes about sexuality that, under the regime of tropical thinking, had initially dismissed the possibility that Asia would ever have its own epidemic.

Between Diaspora and Vector: Perpetual Motion

The early recognition of AIDS in African nonnationals residing in Belgium and France and in Afro-Caribbean nonnationals living in the United States ignited concern over the possibilities of transnational, transcultural exchange of "AIDS." Both the WHO's regional scheme and the emerging pattern scheme had a story to tell about these migrants: They could be either aliens whose infection confirmed the spatiality of the epidemic or heterosexuals who confirmed the temporal dispersion out of the original group. Both stories begged the questions of how and when the virus got from point A to point B, but the spatial story emphasized the traditional routes of travel and their interruption, while the temporal account sought an explanation for the drift of infection between supposedly distinct sexualities. Both accounts were taken up, but

by different agencies. International policy followed its tropical heritage and instituted border restrictions; the GPA
and the International Red Cross used epidemiologic data
to defy national interests in promoting conventional ideas
of sexuality in an effort to understand how sexualities had
been linked—or transformed—in such a way that the virus
could cross the supposedly fixed cordon between homosexuality and heterosexuality.

Many countries at first responded with international
travel restrictions based solely on haphazard stereotypes
about country of origin. (India attempted to deport or exclude African students; the Soviet Union implemented
compulsory testing of everyone staying longer than three
months, but it was chiefly concerned about Americans and
Angolans; the United States used the AIDS panic to
strengthen the case against admitting Haitians.) By 1990,
as many as fifty-five countries, including the United States,
Canada, the United Kingdom, and Australia, had imposed
HIV-related restrictions on incoming travelers, despite
clear policy and human rights statements from the WHO,
the International Red Cross, the United Nations, and the
Council of Europe, which all decried such restrictions
(Cohen and Wiseberg 1990, 36–37). Based on its vast ac-
cumulation of epidemiologic data, the GPA advocated
transnationally administered prevention programs rather
than border controls. It saw border controls based on national origin and fear of infection as human rights viola-
tions, and it also felt such controls hamstrung its transnational authority, since some countries insisted that they
had no epidemic within their national borders.

Although there had been migrants who had AIDS from the earliest case tallies and although this had generated concern about HIV's spatial dimension, serious scientific interest in the role of population mobility in enabling the dispersion of HIV came only after the epidemic made its "late arrival" in Asia. Although the growing body of information on mobility and HIV drew on the traditional, spatially oriented paradigm of migration studies, the data were collected in order to answer epidemiologic questions about the relationship between sexualities. Thus, the difficulties in understanding sexuality, gender, and mobility from the standpoint of global political economy—difficulties that were built into the initial migration-studies paradigm—produced a mismatch between the studies and the need for, in particular, HIV-prevention programs.

For example, there was quite a bit of research about male truckers and male seasonal workers that presented a good description of the men's sexual patterns and identities. However, few of these studies sought to describe the lives of the women they met along the way. Education and policy focused on the "proper" wives and partners the men left behind, ignoring the reality that the women who work at truck stops as sex workers or as hawkers also migrate and also have families situated "at home" elsewhere. The plight of women in developing countries who migrate to cities filled the media and international AIDS information literature of the early 1990s, but it was some years before researchers studied the structure and health implications of this migrational pattern. Unlike media descriptions of migrant men and their regular routes, media descriptions of migrant women portrayed them as poor and uneducated, inhabitants of primordial countrysides who seep into the city, where they are forced into a life of sin. Lost in these images was the reality that female migration in the developing world is an unintended consequence of colonial and postcolonial development plans, whereas male migration, however exploitative, has been planned and is at least partially documented and studied within the formal economy. Women drift out of unacknowledged roles in agriculture and into the undocumented economy of small-scale hawking, temporary unskilled employment, and sex work. Insofar as migration research of the early 1990s considered such women at all, it saw them as uneducable and lost victims at best, threats to orderly development at worst.

Research and policy were slow to respond to the need for new, gender-sensitive concepts because the development schemes and legal structures on which these studies were based—and which they sought to evaluate—were already gender-biased. By virtue of the informal status of female migration, the reality that it makes up a substantial part of the illegal and undocumented economy of both developing and developed countries is almost impossible to quantify. To the extent that the very concept of migration already takes the nation or region as its focus, and given that nations institute normative sexualities through religious ideas and population-control programs, nationally or regionally focused studies of mobility are especially unlikely to capture the dynamics that enabled HIV to make its way around the globe. An individual's chances of contracting HIV do not depend on national identity or regional location as much as on the particular network of mobilities in which he or she is located. Especially in the case of sexual practices perceived as deviant—whether they are homosexualities or sexualities put up for sale—the very networks of identification and transaction are probably obscured from national and regional planners and health controllers.

Furthermore, discussions of migration and sexuality have resulted in a kind of massive outing for people with relatively little power over the representation of their lives. Policy makers and government officials often attempt to join migrants' "other," non-home-state sexualities to the public space of national policy debates, without regard for the local effect of "accusing" migrants of perversions. As I suggested earlier, there was a strong tendency to join the unique sexualities of a particular place to the idea of "the Homosexual" that has been globalized through representations of the epidemic. Countries that belatedly discovered homosexuality within their borders tried to explain it away either as a Western import or as different from and separate from that in the West. When successful, these arguments dismissed the need to produce prevention programs that would aid particular groups of men in the transborder sexual worlds they occupied.

By focusing almost exclusively on cyclical male migration from areas of supposedly low incidence to areas of supposedly high incidence, the dominant form of research on HIV and migration "heterosexualized" and modernized the developing nation. This pattern of migration was thought to increase men's risk of contracting HIV while away from a defined "home," which thereby increased the risk of wives or partners "at home." As if in imitation of the tropical model of the colonists' excursion, the risk of migration was here understood to come from the distant locale, especially from the cities, mining camps, and truck stops, where were found the imagined HIV-saturated commercial sex workers. But there was also a vectoral dimension to these studies: The mobile bodies carried their infection back home to women in rural or semirural areas, who were viewed as ignorant and helpless victims of promiscuous males. In some developing countries, this kind of research intensified efforts to keep men from having sex while they were away, and it presumed there was little to be achieved by promoting safe sex at home. Such educational programs saw sexuality as a translatable property of individuals instead of preparing people to expect new rules and different meanings as they traversed individual and collective sexual landscapes. It was hard for researchers to accept that each locale and each form of sexual relationship has its own rules and its own symbolic value and that these do not respect national borders or national fantasies about hearth and home. Indeed, the mingling of participants from different sexual cultures is more likely to be the norm than the exception. But instead of recognizing the intrinsic mobility of bodies and desires, policy makers became obsessed with sex tourism, a phenomenon that allowed for a partial reconciliation of the two ways of explaining the dispersion of HIV.

Although the tropical model placed too much emphasis on finding the original locale of HIV, it nevertheless provided a notion of context to the vectoral imagination of the epidemiology that had no other means to understand the life conditions of its objects. Unfortunately, social science research on HIV could not move very far from trying, implicitly, to trace the trail of blame. The nascent understanding of the dynamics of population movement that might have improved prevention efforts and care delivery relapsed into the punitive stereotypes about sexuality that finally placed blame squarely on sexual deviants. Fantasizing a world without disease—health for all—allows global health policy to resort to blame, even when it has recognized the permeability of geopolitical borders as blockades to communicable disease. In the context of a new disease of epidemic proportions in which the image of feared populations—homosexuals and black immigrants—initially loomed large, the nationalizing concerns of international relations have won out over the denationalizing voice of global health policy.

Border regulators' confidence in the significance of national borders ignores important economic, political, and cultural factors that underlie mobility, rendering invisible important forms of mobility that will always defy borders. Privileging the nation and the ideas of development that follow from it also missed the reality that sexual norms and even sexual practices are locally specific and even at odds with national sexual ideology. Sex tourism, however problematic as a capitalization of differences in global sexual economies, may only formalize and make intentional what the migrant has accidentally discovered: In crossing space, he or she can be many sexual personae.

CHAPTER 4

A Dying Epidemiology

By 1992, there should have been little doubt that the original categories—indeed, the original framework—for understanding AIDS were no longer useful. What we needed was a radical breakthrough in thinking about the epidemic, perhaps some kind of postmodern research discipline that would resort neither to the palpable but corrupt geopolitical spatialization of tropical thinking, nor to the incorporeal temporalizing of epidemiology. We needed new concepts that would vivify the bodies that were not only geographically mobile but also sexually labile. We needed a way to *feel* our bodies as the disrupters of vectors. Unfortunately, this did not happen. On the contrary: U.S. social scientists and policy makers and the media's translations of their thoughts and policies shifted U.S. thinking about prevention closer to the concepts of tropical medicine that had proved so disastrous in prevention efforts abroad.

I began this book by recalling the rise of AIDS activism in the United States and then slowly made my way through a tour of places and of policies that both rely on and disrupt the two thoughtstyles that I argued are built into scientific and activist concepts of the epidemic. I want to suggest now that tropical ideas are overtaking epidemiologic ideas in the area of AIDS policy, and that this shift in the ground of AIDS thinking has important implications for activists. I am not arguing that activists should try to save the epidemiology that we have contested for more than a decade. I simply want to point out the problems in accepting tropical thinking as the alternate framework. Hopefully, a clearer understanding of how activists have recruited both logics to our advantage will enable us to see the ways in which their extension will eventually prove problematic. As I have shown throughout, the tropical tendencies have always been present in U.S. thinking about the epidemic. Institutionalized in some domains of global policy, these have proven useful. However, activist strategies must now move beyond appropriating and contestating these inherited logics, beyond taking advantage of the strategic opening made possible by playing one against the other. Science changes, and no scientific narrative is ever secure. Activist strategies of the third decade of the epidemic—which opens at the beginning of the twenty-first century—must propose new political and scientific models rather than adapt to the disjunct stories that science, through policy and media, tells.

Tropical States: Ground Zero

On Sunday, 7 March 1993, controversial AIDS-beat journalist Gina Kolata reported on the National Research Council's newly published report "The Social Impact of AIDS." She wrote:

> With AIDS now entrenched in many American cities, some experts are reaching a startling and controversial conclusion. They say the epidemic in the United States can be all but stamped out, even without a vaccine or wonder drug, by prevention efforts that zero in on 25 or 30 hard-hit neighborhoods across the nation.[1]

It appeared that the silence of the Reagan administration and the first Bush administration was over and that the Clinton administration would wake up to the necessity of producing prevention material and programs, even if these might be offensive to those outside the communities in which they had been developed. But veteran AIDS activists, who had for a decade fretted in the face of government unwillingness to support meaningful safe-sex organizing within communities, were skeptical: The "experts'" apparent "discovery" of the value of "messages whose language and imagery were intended for specific neighborhoods" (26) was outrageously late.

Though her story is an unsubtle reading of the report,[2] Kolata performs a shift—tentatively bringing together "community organizing" and "targeting"—that indeed is present in the report. At least for her readers, she hastens the collapse of epidemiology into tropical thinking, a collapse that had been held off for as long as the powerful institution of U.S. epidemiology could subordinate tropical thinking to its own. For the unwary reader, she presents this shift, one immediately linked to plans to "stamp AIDS out," as a major change in scientific thinking, the sort of breaking news that reporters are supposed to discover. However extensive was the shift in U.S. policy—and I think it *was* significant, especially in the CDC's own shift from a rhetoric of community to a rhetoric of targeting—Kolata's story both accelerated and was symptomatic of a shift in how one could secure the scientific referent for the story of AIDS.

As problematic as epidemiology had been, I am not sure the new tropicalizing was a great improvement. The proposed "ground zero" approach to prevention, which focused near-total effort on a small number of hard-hit places thought to represent the chief reservoirs of infection, was no less frightening than the information campaigns proclaiming that "anyone can get AIDS." The latter promoted inaction born of vagueness, but an active campaign "targeting" AIDS could only ever arrive after seroprevalence rates (percentage of a given population calculated to be infected with an agent, here, HIV) were so high that prevention could only mean containment within spaces marked out for destruction. Kolata unwittingly echoes the gay rights slogan "We are everywhere" to re-visualize HIV (and more subtly, homosexuals and drug users) from a mobile and expanding blanket "spread throughout the nation" (1) to a static patchwork of hot spots, "clustered in two of nine [New York City] ZIP codes" (26). Her relocation of HIV from here to there and conflation of disease and bodies enables an implicit but damning shift from "we"—a society with a new disease among us—to "they," who live semicontained, with "their disease," over there. So vivid—and enthusiastically tropical—is Kolata's language that she obscures the larger dispute between scientific theories of the epidemic: epidemiological versus tropical thinking. Kolata achieves her reportorial coup precisely because she adopts the account of science that science likes to have told of itself: Science is not a competition between powerful systems of knowledge for prestige and resources but a neutral endeavor whose breakthroughs produce new truth. Instead of detailing the structure and play of competing thoughtstyles—as I have labored to do here—Kolata claims there is a

new, more effective technique for producing HIV demographics, a technique that has rendered epidemiology as
we have known it unnecessary:

> The new view of the disease's pattern of spread emerged
> from a recent analysis by a committee of the National
> Research Council that suggests AIDS is devastating a
> handful of neighborhoods while leaving most of the
> nation relatively unscathed. (1)

Kolata is not oblivious to the tension among scientists
that the new mapping of domestic AIDS represents. But
her acknowledgment that "others disagree" masks a fundamental refusal to recognize that the issue is power, not
shades of truth. She ignores critics' plaintive cry that this
change in the scientific thoughtstyle will result in radical
and rapid changes in policy.

> The AIDS epidemic "is very rapidly spreading throughout
> smaller and smaller communities each year," said Dr. June
> E. Osborn, chairwoman of the National Commission on
> AIDS. "AIDS sustains itself awfully well. As soon as the
> virus is present, as it now is everywhere, risk-taking
> behavior becomes significant." (26)

In Osborn's account, risk is contingent on viral presence, a drifting territorialization of already-existing behavior—behavior that was once insignificant, safe only
because of viral absence—by an agent that now traces its
course through dispersing spaces of "smaller and smaller
communities." This is the epidemiologic mind at its clear-
est, marking spaces through describable trajectories of
a disease phenomenon, reinventing the meaning of quo-

tidian acts by placing them within a model of transmissibility. What Kolata dismisses is the fateful paradox that is the meat and potatoes of institutionalized epidemiology: Once-innocent or completely unnoticed acts are redescribed as "risk-taking behavior" once a transmissible agent takes advantage of them, an agent that now determines the whole trajectory of an already existing but previously not "significant" conduit. This description, which Kolata reduces to the losing side in a minor disagreement over the meaning of a major breakthrough, highlights the aspect of epidemiology that the mainstream culture finds so troubling. Situating risk as the double inscription of transient presence (repetition and infection) in a chain of transmission erodes the line between "homosexual" and "heterosexual behavior," destroying both the idea that homosexual behavior can be considered risky regardless of the presence of opportunistic microbes and the presumption that heterosexual practices, contained in the safe homeland of heterosexuality, are by definition safe. Kolata herself opts for the reassuring spatiality that defines bodies as separate. But epidemiology knows that any and all bodies can be connected, given the right agent and conditions. *The connection is just a matter of time.*

Kolata's splicing of epidemiologic concepts into a more fundamentally tropical account may appear to be journalistic objectivity; the bulk of her account sides with the "wide variety of experts from a variety of disciplines [who are] urging a tighter focus" (1). But the debate she is describing is less about the "pattern" of "spread" than it is about *which* policy framework should be privileged

in explaining—and now in coping with—the proliferation of HIV during the Reagan-Bush decade of official
nonresponse.

I am not suggesting that either epidemiologic or tropical thinking provides better explanations, affords better
policy, or presents a more appealing object for activism. I
linger over Kolata's account because it is a convenient
place to notice the larger shift in thoughtstyle context in
which local U.S. activism must operate. Focusing on the
surface "debate" obliterates the work of community activists who have toiled for two decades in the face of inaction. The resistant communities formed and protected by
prevention organizing are transformed into "targets" of a
"new" government-sponsored, heat-seeking-missile-like
HIV-prevention program. The locales that appear to be
densely populated by gay men or drug users are now the
objects of prevention, not the sites of agents actively struggling to re-create their world. The competing concepts of
space and movement already embedded within policy discourses switch positions: Tropical ideas predominate and
underwrite a new "solution" to disease, and they promote
new connotations for the basic characters in the story.

Epidemiology's risk groups produced flawed policy
by making it possible for those avoiding prevention messages to say, "I'm not one of *those.*" The tropical model
allows an equally disastrous ignoring of prevention advice:
"I don't live/go there." The dissemination of prevention
advice—so hard to achieve in this epidemic because listen-
ing means admitting being queer—is at two removes; the
reaction is not just "they're not talking to me" but "that
message doesn't belong here." Not only will this distancing

intensify the censorship of the form of safe-sex materials, but it will even more strictly circumscribe where the materials may go—certainly not to schools or on television. But even more depressing, people living with HIV are once again domesticated and isolated, stripped of their public voice. They will not be perceived as an appropriate audience for mass media updates on treatment improvements or policy revisions, nor will they be accepted as valuable prevention advocates. If we as a society continue to desire a "face of AIDS," it will not be to show that we are all basically the same but, rather, to show that those who are already projected as deviants do not live here. The tropical model removes epidemiology's ambivalence about de jure quarantine; prevention becomes a matter of formalizing local, de facto containment rather than a matter of dispersing knowledge about safe sex and safe needle use. Kolata's article graphically registers this shift in perspective:

> The council said the epidemic was "settling into spatially and socially isolated groups and possibly becoming endemic in them." As a result, the committee wrote, "many geographic areas and strata of the population are virtually untouched by the epidemic and probably never will be," while "certain confined areas and populations have been devastated." (1)

The juxtaposition of "the population" and "populations," open "geographic areas and strata" versus "confined areas [that] have been devastated," stakes its self-assurance in ostensive, spatial terms, not performatively self-producing ones. In this increasingly common account, transmission is a function of relative densities of space. In the precise homological form that is the rhetorical strategy of tropical medicine, virus, body, and community stand as homologues for the larger idea of colony:

> [I]f you are going to have sexual transmission outside of infected communities, you need a fairly high rate of contact. The disease can and does break out of the tight communities where it festers, but it cannot sustain itself there, [Dr. Albert Jonsen, an ethics professor at the University of Washington and the chairman of the National Research Council's committee] said. (26)

Substitute "colony," "body," or "virus" for "community": gay men are no longer self-naming; they are simply self-identical. We no longer need to name in order to break the chain of vectoral movement. Infected gay men are already contained by virtue of being tied to a space, the very space of their domestic legibility under capitalism, their ZIP codes: "Within those neighborhoods, the researchers said, H.I.V. infections clustered in two of nine ZIP codes. Gay men who were not part of this community were not infected" (26).

Similarly, though drug users are apparently situated in no particular place, they are also already contained by virtue of their very passivity. Even though they are not visible through their participation in capitalism (survey forms and credit ratings have no means to link their forms of production and consumption to a household), they apparently do not move out of their space:

> The second epidemic in New York involved drug users and their sex partners. There, too, the infections were spread within small local networks of people. Dr. [Shirley] Lindenbaum [City University of New York anthropologist

on the committee] and Dr. [John] Gagnon [State University of New York–Stonybrook sociologist on the committee] wrote that intravenous drug users and their sex partners appeared "to be a relatively immobile population." (26)

Rather than recognizing the gay "community," which has not only reconstituted itself through prevention organizing but has also been the very site of the epidemic's greatest publicity, another medical expert is recruited to Kolata's scheme to reduce resistant queer culture to a colony, a space to which the scientist and policy makers ("we") may go and from which they may return triumphant but un*aff*ected and un*inf*ected: "'If we want to really deal with the epidemic, we have to go where the epidemic is,' said Dr. [Allan] Brandt, a member of the National Research Council's committee" (26).

But what will they do when they get there? That depends on how well activists are able to recognize and resist or capitalize on the securing of space by the emerging tropical discourse. It is urgent to rethink the terrain on which activism occurs, determining whether and how micropractices of resistance can operate in a new land where space, instead of the medical discourse of risk, secures identities.

Since the early 1990s, AIDS activists have battled against epidemiology's misnaming of "risk groups." Although the National Research Council report nods toward the long-sought-after "culturally sensitive" programs, it does so for the wrong reasons. It does not accept June Osborn's description of an epidemic mismanaged and allowed to go "everywhere" because policy makers could not bring themselves to let communities speak for and to

themselves. The report promotes "targeting" out of a conviction that the epidemic has largely stayed in one place.
By thus misunderstanding the epidemic's behavioral dynamics, "targeting" emphasizes cordoning off the "disease" by conflating the virus and the community ideologically constructed in relation to it. Capitalizing on the
anxiety about who is meant to hear safe-sex advice that
epidemiology's emphasis on risk behavior produced, the
tropicalizing move stabilizes as material, as *real*, the erroneous line that divides those who (from a tropical perspective) should attend to the techniques of safer sex and
needle hygiene from those who needn't. Although activists
took full advantage of the window of opportunity that this
shift toward local specificity afforded in terms of funding,
the broader shift in thoughstyle left activists unprepared
for battle against a new, equally problematic discursive
regime that used locality to isolate instead of to educate.

Coda: Back to Africa, Millennium Returns

"Scientists Warn of Inaction as AIDS Spread in China"
(Elisabeth Rosenthal, *New York Times* on the Web,
2 August 2000)

Researchers and medical experts warn that the situation
is worse than a disaster because most disasters have a
foreseeable end. There is none in sight to the advance of
AIDS across Africa. With areas of high population density,
extreme poverty, migrant labor and dysfunctional family
life, South Africa is a microcosm of the way AIDS can
spread and the socioeconomic fallout of the pandemic.
(Hynes, "Fatal Destiny," *New York Times* on the Web,
7 July 2000)

Take a walk down Main Street Africa and the signs of economic decay—poverty, corruption, crime and hopelessness—are all too obvious. (Robinson, "Death Row," 17 July 2000)

The epidemic has hit with devastating force—and things will get much worse before they get better. As a metaphor for hopelessness, it's hard to equal the AIDS crisis in sub-Saharan Africa. (Lemonick, "Little Hope, Less Help," *New York Times* on the Web, 24 July 2000)

One of those risk factors [that excluded blood donors] is male-to-male sex, according to the United States Food and Drug Administration, which regulates the blood supply in the United States and helps set the standards used in much of the world. Others include using intravenous drugs, having sex with prostitutes and traveling in Africa. (Cauvin, "South Africa in a Quandry: Should Gays Donate Blood?" *New York Times* on the Web, 11 June 2000)

Scientists meeting here [Durban, South Africa] debated today what to do about a puzzling but potentially important finding about AIDS: that circumcised men are much less likely to become infected than uncircumcised men.

The finding was first made in Africa more than a decade ago and has been noted in more than 40 studies since then. . . .

No one believes that circumcision, which has been widely and traditionally practiced in Africa, could be the sole explanation of such differences [noted in southern Africa]. Differing rates could be caused by other cultural or religious practices, or by difference in hygiene or other factors. (Altman, "Mystery Factor Is Pondered at AIDS Talk: Circumcision," *New York Times* on the Web, 10 July 2000)

To have lived with H.I.V. for a decade or more is to have
died with it many times over. (Steinhauer, "The New
Landscape of AIDS," *New York Times* on the Web, 25 June
2000)

The rise [in new infections] is deeply troubling because
it was seen in San Francisco, one of the principal centers
of the AIDS epidemic when it was first detected in 1981.
Thus, the rise could signal a new wave of infections there
and elsewhere. (Altman, "H.I.V. Cases Jump in San
Francisco," *New York Times* on the Web, 1 July 2000)[3]

We always tell our students not to quote without explaining, but I'm stopped cold by the echoes in the above
reportage of the Thirteenth International Conference on
AIDS held in Durban in 2000. The disease phenomenon
that since the early 1980s has produced apocalyptic rhetoric from the right and loomed as a spectacular end for so
many individuals and geographical places still lacks a cure,
and the realities of the continued transmission of HIV
remain depressing. As the reportage about the Thirteenth International Conference on AIDS reveals, little
has changed, not even the need to present the known as
the new.

It was incredibly depressing for me to read the coverage of the conference as I labored to put the final touches
on this very much overdue manuscript. This project was
hard to finish, in part because it is located in a much-
contested area of science and society studies, but even
more because genealogical research, as a "history of the
present," is always in reference to the events and problems of the very time in which the researcher is embed-

ded. If the present is drifting under one's feet, then what counts as important, what lines should one follow? Despite the Durban conference's failure to fulfill any of its promise—as a "first conference" in a developing country, as a moment of cultural exchange among scientists, as a way station from which to measure the progress of medical understanding, even as a forum to air political grievances about the pandemic's management—the extent to which the reportage forgot the past and yet echoed, as if no time had passed at all, the conceptual problems of defining and addressing an epidemic—problems I see as epistemic—suggests that my genealogy has merit. Though I wish I were writing "the end" of the epidemic, I too am still rewriting its beginning: a disease lodged ineluctably *here*, an epidemic that remains more future than past.

Of course, some important changes occurred during the 1990s: the advent of the "cocktail," or highly active antiretroviral treatment (HAART), and its seeming acceptance as reliable amelioration of the problem of HIV; the shifting of the "face of AIDS" toward developing countries and poor communities within the developed world; the folding of the GPA into UNAIDS, a project much more like the long-standing intersectoral programs that have long characterized the WHO's structure. But these changes have not challenged the basic framework I have laid out here. In fact, in several cases, these changes can be explained in terms of the drift between the tropical and epidemiologic thoughtstyles. I want to briefly outline these relationships, with reference to the representation of the Thirteenth International Conference on AIDS.

Lost Cure

The state of drug therapy was debated on two fronts in the summer of 2000. The optimism of 1992's early success with HAART has faded, not only because only a modest number of those who can even get the drug combinations actually benefit, but also because studies of those who remain on them for many years now show that the regimes are exhausting to many treatment subjects. Living with HIV gave way to living with the side effects and restrictions on daily life imposed by the multidose therapeutic regimes. Those who perceived HAART as a miracle cure, or as a sign that the epidemic no longer had bite because it was "easy" to stop an infection, had not yet considered what it might be like to be shackled to the treatment regimes: better than the threat of imminent death, but no kind of life either.

But for the First World poor and for any but the very, very richest members of poor countries, there remained another problem with treatments: cost. Modest breakthroughs, at least on the political level, occurred in relation to the just distribution of medical resources, breakthroughs importantly indebted to the work of ACT UP Philadelphia, one of the most multicultural and diverse health activist groups in the world. Members of the group took the lead in challenging presidential candidate Al Gore—and thereby the Clinton administration—to stand in solidarity with developing countries and European advocates who were trying to pressure drug companies to lower the cost of treatments not only of HAART but also, and much more importantly, of the more common drugs that fight the opportunistic infections associated with

HIV. The dramatic differences in morbidity and mortality of HIV between developed and developing countries is largely due to the virtual unavailability of the drugs that since the late 1980s have prolonged the lives and increased the comfort of the infected in developed countries. Also forcing this change in drug distribution was the fact that Thailand and South Africa decided to ignore international agreements and trade norms and manufacture generic versions of several HIV spectrum drugs. Fearing a loss of market, several companies have initiated discount programs, and there continues to be pressure on drug companies to make public the formula for drugs in order to speed up their release in developing countries that could make the drugs on their own. In addition to the faint promise of at least getting some drugs to people who need them, the shift in political discourse is extremely significant: Activists are now operating on the world stage and challenging international drug policy and global distribution practices. Contesting the tropical discourse that suggests that "Africa"—and now by extension, any resource-poor country—is lost, salvageable only by the hoped-for vaccine (what happened to the "vaccine of education"?), activists argue instead for concrete intervention for the sick: treatment, not containment.

The Other Changing Face of AIDS

Since the beginning of the epidemic, we have been told that the "face of AIDS" is changing. One wonders if the "face" has ever been "the same." The epidemic's first face-lift entailed convincing Americans that "anyone can get AIDS"—that the "face" was not marked queer, was in fact not marked at all. That face changed quickly: white, straight, Middle America never believed that its members could "get AIDS," so the "everyone" quickly transformed into "everyone but me," making the face of AIDS, now represented through full bodies, more plural but also more concretely marked: black, brown, gay, prostitute.

This new face change, or maybe we should say change of face, marks developing *countries*, symbolized by and as Africa, as those persons who are to be seen as the embodiment of an epidemic. Now, ominously, the face is continents and countries, not stereotypes of risky people. The sense of who is dangerous has changed from the standpoint of global representation, even if on the local level, the masks of risk still cover the faces of those most affected by the epidemic. But here again, two larger conceptions of the disease phenomenon coexist in different dimensions of space and with different regulating bodies: the face in or of Africa, and several faces of "Risky People" who scatter across the globe.

Folding AIDS into World Health

The final and most significant change of the 1990s concerns the global management of HIV. The GPA was ultimately merged with other programs serving related needs among those especially affected by AIDS. This multisectoral approach had the potential to maximize the money and energy directed toward such problems as orphans and poverty and HIV, or women and migration and HIV or any of many other additive functions. But this approach has failed on two fronts. First, it did not actually direct any more resources to poor countries and places (the In-

ternational Monetary Fund and World Bank did more—
and with more politically devastating effects—when they
decided to offset debt by returning interest with AIDS
dollars; see Parker 1999). But second, by losing the distinction between microscopic virus and macroeconomic
processes, the groundwork was laid for HIV-dissidents
(those who contest the HIV-AIDS connection) to gain
scientific credibility for an ill-argued claim that poverty
(as if that were a single thing) is the cause of AIDS. This
played out devastatingly right at the opening of the Thirteenth International Conference on AIDS when President Thabo Mbeki refused to discount the theories of the
HIV-dissident scientists he had consulted. Over the course
of the conference, it became clear that Mbeki was trying
to point out the significance of health care infrastructure
and the social and medical effects of poverty on AIDS as
a disease process and epidemic, but the damage had already been done. Playing into the space where epidemiology and tropical thinking collapse, Mbeki widened the
possibilities for seeing Africa and developing countries as
places that are lost because they are too poor to be saved
rather than as places that urgently need more community
organizing, more health care funding, more access to drugs,
and more creative use of treatment.

Replacing the Epidemic

I do not want to leave this volume on a note of hopelessness. But indeed, the role of broad systems of medical
thought in framing our understanding of our bodies and
our places in the HIV pandemic is large. There is no "outside" to scientific thought. A brilliant series of cascading

representations, science is made of the best thought of our day, even as it reshapes our vision of the physically possible. The way ahead is one that joins the work of science, in its many registers and modes, with the political sensibilities that have arisen from critical analyses of science, of politics, and of experience. For many of us, "AIDS" has now long been and may always be the defining experience of our time. But the paradoxes, tragedies, and frustrations that have marked our time and our place also connect us to many other world-epoch-defining experiences, and these links are forged on the tracks of the major thoughtstyles I have tried to characterize here.

Notes

Introduction

1. The test that is colloquially called an "AIDS test" actually tests for the antibody to human immunodeficiency virus, or HIV, the agent most scientists believe is the decisive factor distinguishing AIDS from other immune disorders. Border restrictions were proposed for homosexuals, hemophiliacs, Haitians, and prostitutes even before a virus was associated with AIDS. Execution of such an exclusion scheme would have been difficult but neither impossible nor unprecedented; indeed, the United States already included homosexuals among those who could be excluded from the United States for reasons of public health.

This test (there are several varieties with different levels of accuracy)—and more sophisticated confirmatory tests that actually "read" the virus itself—is now commonly and widely in use. But in the four years from first recognition of cases to the discovery of an agent to the development of a reliable test and the implementation of ethical and coherent counseling programs to accompany mass public testing was a long, long time. There was considerable dispute about whether the "right virus" had been found, much less what the sequence of clinical developments would be. Indeed, in an important sense, the test and the disease's definition are tautological: Scientists needed a test to distinguish this immune system failure from others—especially in poor countries where debilitating malaise is common— in order to understand more clearly the progression of HIV-related disease. The clinical uncertainty about the cause of AIDS and the significance of other factors, as well as the lack of any clear treatments, made the value of the test to the individual unclear. In addition, health educators early and insistently believed that knowing that one was positive would prompt behavior change among the infected, and even for those who tested negative, the terror of waiting for the result would inspire a change away from risky behavior. I have written more extensively on the social impact of the test in my *Inventing AIDS* (1990) and *Fatal Advice* (1996).

2. In the process of identifying what is now called HIV, scientists from several laboratories around the world characterized the genetic code of viral material suspected to be the cause of AIDS. There were always differences among these isolates; however, the differences did not seem to correlate statistically to different expressions of AIDS. By the late 1980s, there was sufficient evidence of a cluster of cases in western Africa, all with the same pattern of genetic difference; later, another cluster was found in Southeast Asia. These clusters enabled scientists to begin calculating the mutation rate of HIV and to draw some rough conclusions about the extent to which variants indicated relative closed infection loops versus places where novel variants appeared. None of the isolates seem to suggest a particularly different course of disease, for example, as do the differences among types of hepatitis. However, with the advent of protease inhibitors, and with concern that strains were developing resistance to particular drugs, physicians have been able to use the viral strain characterization to predict more accurately what combination of antiviral drugs a given patient will most likely respond well to.

This is still very far from any ability to claim that any particular strain is a super-viral version of HIV.

3. Although it is cumbersome and has recently fallen out of usage, I have here preferred the term "person *living* with" AIDS or HIV to "person with" AIDS or HIV. The insertion of "living" was crucial to activist politics of the late 1980s and indicated that those who "had" the virus were "living with it" rather than dying from it. In this era of highly publicized success with drug regimes, at least for a lucky but substantial minority of Westerners, the rhetorical importance of asserting the "living with" has diminished.

4. During my years at Emory University there were several cross-departmental initiatives to study emerging illness and communities of suffering. Many faculty members and students, as well as participants in activist communities, have examined the development, impact, and possible role of new illnesses and new ways of thinking about them. Situated down the street from the Centers for Disease Control, a partner in these efforts to bring together disciplinary and popular knowledges of disease, we had access to cutting-edge epidemiology and also, perhaps, had a small role in reshaping the possibilities for including nonscientific disciplines in a rethinking of society and medicine.

1. Critical Bodies

1. By distinguishing two waves of activism, I mean to acknowledge both the organizing activities begun in the early years and now precariously institutionalized at the margins of formal public health systems, and the agitprop activism whose most obvious proponent is ACT UP.

2. Many clinicians and researchers consider HIV to be a "spectrum" disease; that is, there are a range of manifestations of different degrees of severity. Early in the epidemic, different researchers proposed different ways of classifying what was then an emergent phenomenon. There has long been a clinical term to describe persistent swollen lymph nodes: lymphadenopathy. Patients who seemed to fit the profile for AIDS diagnosis but who were not especially sick were initially said to have "AIDS-related lymphadanoplogy," or later, "AIDS-related complex" (ARC). Walter Reed Hospital, the main center for the U.S. Army's medical research, defined a series of stages for the progression for AIDS. Obviously, once a virus was associated with the wide range of illnesses, the idea of an AIDS-related complex became so diffuse as to lose any clinical meaning. As clinicians got more experience with the development of symptoms, they began to realize there was no clear-cut symptomatic progression: Individuals might go through incremental stages of immune system decline, or they might go from very healthy to dead in a short period of time. Thus, the idea of HIV as a spectrum of symptoms, which might or might not progress in a particular sequence, became the popular clinical understanding of the disease. This corresponded well with PLWAs' experience of living with and managing the range of different ailments that befell them. Into the second decade of the epidemic, and especially once the most dramatic symptoms—for example, PCP—could be controlled with drugs, clinicians and PLWAs alike began to rely on things like T-cell counts, rather than subjective symptoms, to gauge how far along viral destruction of the immune system had progressed. This shifting sand of definition was further complicated by the pressure from disability and health insurers, who wanted clear guidelines for who should be covered under their programs. Activists entered the fray in contradictory ways, seeking more rapid research on drug treatments, which might be aided by strict clinical definitions, but also seeking to expand the definitions of AIDS to include more, rather than fewer, affected people in social programs.

3. Early definitions of a new disease are often too restrictive, since epidemiologists are trying to distinguish the most clear-cut examples of a new phenomenon from instances of other known diseases. It is especially difficult to craft definitions when the clinical symptoms used to characterize a new disease phenomenon are vague, overlap those of many other diseases, or are themselves diseases. If an etiologic agent or environmental cause is ultimately found, testing or contact factors are used to distinguish between diseases whose clinical presentation may be similar. For example, viral tests eventually made it possible to distinguish between various types of hepatitis. In the context of HIV, tuberculosis (TB) is a disease in its own right, with a specific bacterial cause. TB is also an opportunistic disease associated with HIV infection. Many people with an average CD4 count might fight the disease off, or they may have relatively undramatic symptoms, compared to a person with HIV and a low CD4 count. This individual might rapidly succumb. From a clinical standpoint, does a person with TB but unknown HIV status have TB or AIDS? If the person tests positive for HIV, he or she will be said to have AIDS, with TB as a symptom.

The original 1982 definition of AIDS was purely clinical, since an etiologic agent had only been hypothesized; indeed, many scientists argued that the new syndrome resulted from environmental or lifestyle factors. During this period of dispute about the actual cause of the syndrome, the term "AIDS" was used only for cases involving the occurrence of Kaposi's sarcoma, *Pneumocystis carinii* pneumonia, or one of a proliferating number of uncommon infections called "opportunistic infections" to indicate that their appearance in the "previously healthy" person was due to an immune-system malfunction. Once a virus was identified and strongly associated with AIDS, both scientists and activists pushed to have the syndrome reconceptualized as HIV disease, which would have a spectrum of manifestations ranging from those an individual actually experienced (the night sweats and malaise, prodromes, i.e., early signs that the body is reacting to an insult) to the secondary diseases of "full-blown" AIDS, to the subclinical changes that could only be identified through monitoring blood chemistry. This idea was only partially accepted: Researchers now recognize stages, but these are still primarily oriented in relation to the original AIDS definition and the concepts it embodied. Activists in the United States have largely focused their efforts on expanding the original case definition to include dramatic symptoms experienced by people living with HIV who fall outside the original conception of the probable client population, that is, those experienced by women, by people who have not had adequate access to health care, by drug injectors, and so on.

4. Lyotard is discussing cases of wrong in which there is a gap between what the parties to the wrong (the doer and the wronged) perceive to be moral. As he puts it, "As distinguished from a litigation, a differend *[différend]* would be a case of conflict, between (at least) two parties, that cannot be equitably resolved for lack of a rule of judgment applicable to both arguments. One side's legitimacy does not imply the other's lack of legitimacy. However, applying a single rule of judgment to both in order to settle their differend as though it were merely a litigation would wrong (at least) one of them (and both of them if neither side admits this rule). Damages result from an injury which is inflicted upon the rules of a genre of discourse but which is reparable according to those rules. A wrong results from the fact that the rules of the genre of discourse by which one judges are not those of the judged genre or genres of discourse" (1988, xi). For Lyotard, a difference of judgment is not an abstraction; rather, it is a concrete situation indicating a lack of a larger rule or agreement about the wrong under discussion. I am suggesting that the first people living with AIDS fought to establish an approximate agreement about the nature of the wrong done to them, although the use of the Kubler-Ross-type narrative I discuss later in the text is, I believe, still inadequate to express their trauma.

5. My invocation of The Name is an oblique reference to the same concept Lyotard developed: Lyotard argues that proper nouns arise from their special use in relation to many contexts. Thus, a proper noun will always partially invoke that universe of meaning, that history of use, and they will carry as a shadow the exclusions that were required to restrict the proper from the general noun. For this section, then, I mean to remind the reader of the contingency and complexity that was stabilized and simplified when myriad experiences and propositions about illness and death and about social deviance and marginality were encapsulated in the proper noun, AIDS.

I also want to acknowledge that there were several earlier names for what we call AIDS: gay bowel syndrome, gay-related immunodeficiency (GRID), and gay cancer. These names were also incorporated in the connotative meaning of AIDS, even if few today remember that they were actually used for brief periods early in the epidemic.

6. I have borrowed this term from Ludwig Fleck, the early-twentieth-century laboratory scientist whose theoretical work *Genesis and Development of a Scientific Fact* has become highly influential among a handful of renegade thinkers, notably, Mary Douglas, especially in her *How Institutions Think* (1986), and Bruno Latour and Steve Woolgar, in their *Laboratory Life* (1979). The term "thoughtstyle" conveys the idea that scientific thinking occurs in a complex milieu composed of the scientist's expert ("esoteric") and common ("exoteric") knowledge. These combine with specialized knowledge formally unrelated to science to produce unpredictable ways of working through problems; for example, a scientist's knowledge of piano may influence her understanding of how an immune system works, or she may use logics drawn from her scientific training to think about everyday problems in her relationships.

Thoughtstyles, then, are an abstraction, indicating the general logic scientists use, with its core of a common academic training, less hegemonic social knowledges, and the very diverse specialized knowledges that individual scientists unknowingly import into the supposedly pristine domain of scientific thought.

7. In fact, there is a much longer history of imagining queer nations than the Queer Nation agitators seemed to realize. For example, Jill Johnston titled a 1973 book *Lesbian Nation*. Henry Abelove (1993) has pointed out the crypto-queerness of Henry David Thoreau's *Walden* and the convergence of identitarian and sexual politics in New Left thinking and ego psychology. Robert Caserio (1997a, 1997b) has elaborated the concepts of citizenship in early-twentieth-century British and U.S. homosexual writings.

8. "Fag hag," a once-derogatory phrase applied to women who liked to hang out with gay men, was reclaimed in the 1980s, as gay identities and the word "fag" were themselves reclaimed. The notion of fag-haggery refers to the general acceptance of strong friendships between men occupying homosexual social roles (hairdressers, florists, ministers in some places) and the women who rely on their services. Even a cursory glance at television or popular films reveals the cultural narrative in which straight men remain unthreatened by relationships between their female partners and other men only because those men are presumed gay. Indeed, it would seem that straight men rely on such bonds to take some of the pressure to "relate" off themselves. It has long interested me that straight men largely put up with their female partners' interest in AIDS volunteer work: Straight women (not least, Liz Taylor) could become deeply involved with care and activism because there was no apparent threat that they would become infected (since they would not be having sex with these men).

9. There are many competing theories of what social movements are and how they work. In one model, there is an actual reality that government or society has obscured through ideology. Unmasking this ideology is a matter of pointing out the "lies" promulgated by government or society. The other main model argues that movements construct themselves as they go along, helping people reframe their identities in order to become the agents of their own destinies. Although any movement is a contradictory mix of reality-claiming and reality-producing, ACT UP tended more toward the latter. Thus, although they made rhetorical use of the concept of "lie!"—indeed, they often made posters and chanted slogans specifying who was lying about what—they meant this with a sense of irony. They were destabilizing socially or governmentally produced ideas—for example, that AIDS was under control, and hence, Ronald Reagan did not really need to say the word—by accusing politicians of lying. They hoped that by narrowing the space for deniability, they could actually force government to act in new ways, such as speeding up drug-trial procedures. For ACT UP, then, neither lies nor truths were fixed realities; rather, both were markers for broader patterns of action. This is in sharp contrast to more conventional social movements' strategies, in which "new information" is offered to counter "lies" as if the power of the newly uncovered truth is sufficient to cause politicians to change their actions.

2. From Colonial Medicine to World Health

1. On one hand, the wealthy nations should pay for such global efforts. But on the other hand, this gives them undue influence, especially in the case of the U.S. grip on the entire region of the Americas, where PAHO, administered from Washington, D.C., operates virtually autonomously from the rest of the WHO. In fact, such control may mean that the highly developed countries receive indirect benefits out of proportion to their contributions. The WHO's smallpox program, for example, cleaned up the mess made by European and American colonial and imperial schemes that actively or passively introduced the disease into vast areas of the globe. Without discounting the Third World lives saved, it is also true that eradicating smallpox from the Third World (it had been eradicated from the developed world decades earlier) clearly made international travel and conscription of poor workers across borders a much less risky proposition for people from developed countries. Perhaps the developed countries should pay even more.

2. Epidemiology emerged late in the history of modern medicine, probably sometime in the early nineteenth century with the establishment and acceptance of germ theory. The ideas that disease was simply a reflection of God's will, inherent degeneracy among certain types of people, or witchcraft had to subside before epidemiologists could develop contact models for the dispersion of disease, which in turn required them to obtain answers from the afflicted that corresponded closely enough to their own theories of disease. For example, even if the epidemiologist hypothesized a transmissible germ, if afflicted persons insisted they were victims of witchcraft and refused to say whom they had seen and where they had been, epidemiologists could not do their work. The social acceptance of germ theory was slower than the disciplinary acceptance of epidemiologic modeling, so it was convenient if public health officers could have overall ideas of who might fall sick from certain types of ailment, even if popular understandings of cause differed from medical models. Cholera proved to be an excellent case in which to develop epidemiologic surveillance: Because cholera in the nineteenth century was spread through the merchant marine, it turned out that prostitutes serving the waterfront were the first visible evidence of an emergent cholera epidemic. The sailors often moved on before their own illness was widely recognized, but the prostitutes remained as a group in one place. Thus, epidemiologists developed the idea of "sentinels" or groups who would evidence an epidemic first (even if they were not the first cases). Sentinel studies, then, are prospective studies of population groups that epidemiologists believe will show dramatic increases in a disease in advance of large numbers of more dispersed cases. Prostitutes continue to be "sentinels" for STD surveillance, but any group of individuals who are easy to track and likely to be hard hit by an arriving epidemic disease that is predicted to spread to a "general population" would qualify as "sentinels" for study purposes. For example, a group of seniors who mall-walk every morning might be good sentinels for influenza prediction. People who eat nightly at fast-food hamburger joints could be studied to monitor *E. coli* bacteria outbreaks.

3. By the late 1990s, *becoming quarantined* no longer required confinement in asylum or home. The epidemiology-based understanding of condom use, although contested and reworked by progressives working to promote safe-sex practices was finally *experienced* by many gay men as a kind of quarantine. This may be part of the source of the "barebacking" movement that, at least among those who make a liberatory political project of it, seems to be an effort to resist quarantine at the most intimate level. Heather Worth's analysis of Australian and New Zealander safe-sex projects points to the cultural constructedness of what she called "semen essentialism," that is, the deeply felt conviction that semen and its exchange is psychically fundamental to gay men's sense of self. She suggests that this construction unwittingly works in tandem with the public health safe-sex campaigns, which many gay men experience as an attack on their most fundamental desires. By locating both the sense that one is being attacked for one's way of life and one's means of resistance to that attack in a supposedly intransigent desire, men put themselves at risk of viral transfer at the moment they try to rescue themselves through deep sexual communion. I suggest that "semen essentialist" thinking rejects the idea of containment (from epidemiology) in favor of an idea of group embedded in space. By contesting condoms—and at the deep level of psychic constitution—and the epidemiologic thinking that underwrites their use in safe sex, the organized resistance to conventional understandings of safe sex seen, for example, in the political expressions of "barebackers," constructs a tribe-like space more consistent with the tropical model of who might harbor disease. "Barebacking," and the general neo-tribalism of urban American subcultures of the 1990s, may be more like the subaltern of the colony: resisting through a mimicry that is inadvertently self-annihilating.

4. There was ongoing debate about whether the gay men from the San Francisco hepatitis B prospective study of the late 1970s, who became the most significant single database for AIDS epidemiology of the 1980s, should be "allowed" to take AZT and other prophylactic anti–opportunistic infection drugs. I and others observed a heated interchange on the question at an international AIDS conference. To our stunned disbelief, well-known researchers lamented the loss of information about the natural course of HIV that would result if the last remaining asymptomatic and untreated men were to go on HIV treatment regimes. Worse yet, they were interested in seeing how long it would take the men to "finally" get sick, not in studying them in order to find out why they were able to combat the symptoms. The idea of studying the infected as "well" seemed to occur only as an afterthought. And in any case, such studies are not the usual domain of epidemiology, which studies illness patterns, not health patterns. Of course, I would be remiss not to mention the most significant known case of "letting the disease go" in order to find out what would happen: the Tuskegee study of syphilis in black men, conducted continuously (and in full view of medical researchers, because results were intermittently published in reputable journals) from the 1920s through the late 1970s. I do not want to single out epidemiology for its malfeasances; science usually goes wrong because the social order has gone wrong before it, or rather, because social ideologies are *already embedded within* scientific thoughtstyles. My point here is to identify the tendencies in this way of thinking in order to understand what kinds of social and political and scientific ideas epidemiology can be made to support.

5. When the late Jonathan Mann, first head of the Global Programme on AIDS, left his post in 1992, Michael Merson, a career WHO administrator, took his place and began the slow process of bringing the GPA in line with other branches of the WHO.

3. Official Maps

1. Condoms are highly problematic because they are associated with earlier eugenics campaigns waged under the guise of family planning. Disassociating the condom from family planning in order to let it be read as a means of disease prevention has been extremely difficult.

2. "Multiculturalism" has a rather different meaning in Australian English than in contemporary U.S. usage. Australia's originally exclusionary immigrant policy was somewhat liberalized in the 1980s, and multiculturalism emerged as a paradigm for sustaining a nation in the face of radical ethnic difference. Of course, because Aboriginals are not immigrants, they have only recently become part of Australia's vision of a multicultural society. And, somewhat like the First Nations in North America, the Aboriginal peoples of Australia are not so sure they want to erase the history of their brutal displacement in order to be included as only one among many cultures occupying what they view as rightfully their land.

3. I am suggesting that safe-sex practices arose and were globalized as a penalty. For a longer discussion of the rise of prevention discourse, see my *Fatal Advice* (1996).

4. I date this aspect of current gay and lesbian movements to the homophile efforts of the 1950s, since this work with health and educational professionals seems most directly to have resulted in changes in professionals' attitudes, as opposed to in the attitudes of the general public.

5. For example, in the United States and Europe, the existence of massive educational efforts has been used to argue that gay men and prostitutes should recognize their status as members of risk groups. However, because of the conflation of risk groups—people likely to contract a given illness—and stereotypes about levels of sexual deviancy, the "general public" presumes all members of both groups to be already infected and to be putting others at risk. This logic has made criminalization of sex acts extremely appealing. Combined with queer bashers' long-standing self-justification—that they were defending their heterosexuality—this presumption figured importantly in a highly publicized trial in which a hitchhiker who beat two gay men to death pleaded self-defense against the alleged flirtations. Uncertain whether to allow the link between an offer of sex and HIV, the judge finally allowed posthumously obtained evidence of the two victims' serostatuses to be admitted: One was positive, and one negative. However, this was not interpreted to mean that the association of gay looks with seropositivity is false. Rather, it reinforced the idea that the perpetrator had been justified in his fears of infection. In the case's logic, the odds that a gay man is seropositive is a sobering fifty-fifty. Never mind that the defense offered no evidence that the men had or even intended to have sex with the man who murdered them. Although the hitchhiker was convicted of murder, the fact that serostatus, much less sexuality, was an issue nearly overrode two decades of careful work by lawyers and activists to get courts to recognize queer bashing and antigay speech as hate-motivated crimes.

6. The other major global effort to cope with HIV came out of the maternal- and child-health branch of the WHO, an effort that was an equally problematic reduction of women's needs to those relating to childbearing and rearing.

7. The data on probable paths of transmission in the early studies done in Africa are totally unreliable precisely because researchers did not understand the complexity and range of barter relations. If men had ever obtained any kind of sexual favor from a woman, researchers were content to conclude that transmission had resulted from heterosexual sex.

8. The negligible number of cases in the United States attributed to female-to-male transmission and the theoretical difficulty of female-to-male transmission raised the question of why there seemed to be so many such cases in Africa. Instead of reconsidering the heterosexuality of the men under study or more rigorously investigating blood products, scientists hypothesized, though without any data, perverted practices, from male aggressiveness to female douching. None of these alone can account for the gender distribution of cases. The lack of evidence for female-to-male transmission in the United States or Africa has never diminished the attacks on female prostitutes.

9. As I have argued at length elsewhere (Patton 1990), it is by no means clear whether a vaccine is possible, or what "vaccine" even means in the context of a new syndrome whose very definition is still at issue. Some researchers consider early—virtually prophylactic—use of antivirals among health workers who have suffered potentially infectious needlesticks to be a vaccine, blurring the line between vaccine and treatment. Others conceptualize "vaccination" as somehow trapping HIV within infected cells, which are then prevented from reproducing. Recently, infants have been studied to discover whether they "throw off" infections as they develop their own immune systems. (Infants function with the vestiges of their mothers' immune systems until they are about eighteen months old.) Again, the baby-body process is conceived by some researchers as a "natural" immunity that might yield a means of producing vaccination. Whatever potentially exciting work is underway, there is no consensus on the theory, much less the development, of a vaccine for a retrovirus and cofactor complex. Numerous approaches are currently under investigation, but if a vaccine is discovered, it will, like most past vaccines, be discovered more or less by a stroke of scientific good luck. If a vaccine does become available, it will in turn force a scientific and policy reconstruction of what we now know as "AIDS."

4. A Dying Epidemiology

1. Gina Kolata, "Targeting Urged in Attack on AIDS," *New York Times*, 7 March 1993, 1. Page numbers for further quotations appear in parentheses after the citations.

2. I want to make clear at the outset that I am analyzing Kolata's construction of a story and her use of various kinds of "experts" as markers for larger positions and ideas in policy discourse. Indeed, I can imagine that many of the people cited in this particular article were horrified at the role they were made to play as characters in a dispute. I have met or followed the careers of several of those who were quoted by Kolata, and based on my knowledge of those individuals' longtime commitments and activities in policy debate, I believe their quotations are so radically decontextualized as to make them appear to say nearly the opposites of the positions the speakers might actually have taken.

3. All accessed 20 September 2000 at www.nytimes.com.

Abbreviations

ACT UP	AIDS Coalition to Unleash Power
ARC	AIDS-related complex
ASO	AIDS service organization
CDC	Centers for Disease Control
GMHC	Gay Men's Health Crisis
GPA	Global Programme on AIDS
GRID	Gay-related immunodeficiency
HAART	Highly active anti-retroviral treatment
HBO	Home Box Office
MSM	men who have sex with men
NAFTA	North American Free Trade Agreement
NGO	nongovernmental organization
PAHO	Pan American Health Organization
PLWA	people living with AIDS
STD	sexually transmitted disease
TASO	The AIDS Service Organization (Uganda)
UNAIDS	United Nations Joint Program on HIV/AIDS
WHO	World Health Organization

Bibliography

Abelove, Henry. 1993. "From Thoreau to Queer Politic." *Yale Journal of Criticism* 6, no. 2: 17–28.

Abramson, Paul R., and Gilbert Herdt. 1990. "The Assessment of Sexual Practices Related to the Transmission of AIDS: A Global Perspective." *Journal of Sex Research* 27, no. 2 (May): 215–32.

ACT UP NY Women and AIDS Book Group. 1992. *Women, AIDS, and Activism.* Boston: South End Press.

"The AIDS Conflict." 1985. *Newsweek*, 23 September.

Alexander, Nancy J., Henry. L. Gabelnick, and Jeffrey M. Spieler. 1990. *Heterosexual Transmission of AIDS.* New York: Wiley-Liss.

Anderson, J., et al. 1989. "Knowledge of HIV Serostatus and Pregnancy Decisions." Paper presented at the Fifth International Conference on AIDS, 4–9 June, Montreal.

Ankrah, Maxine, et al. 1992. "Rural and Urban Mobility and Attendant Sexual Behavior." Paper presented at the Eighth International Conference on AIDS, 19–24 July, Amsterdam.

Bailey, Patricia, et al. 1992. "Heterogeneity among Commercial Sex Workers and Commonalities of Condom Use." Paper presented at the Eighth International Conference on AIDS, 19–24 July, Amsterdam.

Bernard, Marina, and Neil McKeganey. 1992. "Risk Behaviors among a Sample of Male Clients of Female Prostitutes." Paper presented at the Eighth International Conference on AIDS, 19–24 July, Amsterdam.

Bevier, Pamela, et al. 1992. "Women Who Have Sex with Women and Multiple Risks for HIV at a New York City STD Clinic." Paper presented at the Eighth International Conference on AIDS, 19–24 July, Amsterdam.

Boue, François, et al. 1990. "Risks for HIV-1 Perinatal Transmission Vary with the Mother's Stage of Infection." Paper presented at the Sixth International Conference on AIDS, 20–24 June, San Francisco.

Branch for the Advancement of Women. 1989. "AIDS and Its Effects on the Advancement of Women." In *Women 2000.* Vienna: Centre for Social Development and Humanitarian Concerns.

Brandt, Allan. 1985. *No Magic Bullet.* London: Oxford University Press.

British Voice. 1988. Untitled pamphlet. Hand circulated.

Brockett, Linda, et al. 1992. "HIV/AIDS Prevention Targeting Asian Prostitution in Sydney: A Cultural Perspective." Paper presented at the Eighth International Conference on AIDS, 19–24 July, Amsterdam.

Bronfman, Mario, and N. Minella. 1992. "Sexual Habits of Temporary Mexican-Migrants to the United States of America: Risk Practices for HIV Infection." Paper presented at the Eighth International Conference on AIDS, 19–24 July, Amsterdam.

Campbell, Carole A. 1991. "Prostitution, AIDS, and Preventive Health Behavior." *Social Science and Medicine* 32, no. 12: 1367–78.

Campbell, Ian D., and Glen Williams. 1990. *AIDS Management: An Integrated Approach*. Strategies for Hope Series, no. 3. London: ACTIONAIDS.

Caserio, Robert. 1997a. "Auden's New Citizenship." *Raritan: A Quarterly Review* 17, no. 2: 90–103.

———. 1997b. "Queer Passions, Queer Citizenship: Some Novels about the State of the American Nation, 1946–1954." *Modern Fiction Studies* 43, no. 1: 170–205.

Center for Women Policy Studies. 1990. *The Guide to Resources on Women and AIDS*. Washington, D.C.: Center for Women.

Centers for Disease Control (CDC). 1981a. "Kaposi's Sarcoma and *Pneumocystis* Pneumonia among Homosexual Men—New York City and California." *Morbidity and Mortality Weekly Report* 30, no. 25 (3 July): 305–8.

———. 1981b. "Follow-Up on Kaposi's Sarcoma and *Pneumocystis* Pneumonia." *Morbidity and Mortality Weekly Report* 30, no. 33 (28 August): 431–35.

———. 1982. "Update on Kaposi's Sarcoma and Opportunistic Infections in Previously Healthy Persons—United States." *Morbidity and Mortality Weekly Report* 31, no. 22 (11 June): 294, 300–301.

———. 1983. "Immunodeficiency among Female Sexual Partners of Males with Acquired Immune Deficiency Syndrome (AIDS)—New York." *Morbidity and Mortality Weekly Report* 31, no. 52 (7 January): 697–98.

———. 1987. "Antibody to Human Immunodeficiency Virus in Female Prostitutes." *Morbidity and Mortality Weekly Report* 36, no. 11 (27 March): 157–61.

Chu, Susan, et al. 1990. "Epidemiology of Reported Cases of AIDS in Lesbians, United States, 1980–89." *American Journal of Public Health*.

Cohen, Judith, Pamela Derish, and Mike Swent. 1992. "Different Types of Prostitution Show Wide Variation in HIV and Other Sexually-Transmitted Disease Risk." Paper presented at the Eighth International Conference on AIDS, 19–24 July, Amsterdam.

Cohen, Roberta, and Laurie S. Wiseberg. 1990. *Double Jeapordy—Threat to Life and Human Rights: Discrimination against Persons with AIDS*. Cambridge, Mass.: Human Rights Internet.

Coleman, Samuel. 1981. "The Cultural Context of Condom Use in Japan." *Studies in Family Planning* 12, no. 1 (January): 28–39.

Cowan, Jane E., et al. 1990. "Reproductive Choices of Women at Risk of HIV Infection." Paper presented at the Sixth International Conference on AIDS, 20–24 June, San Francisco.

Day, Sophie, et al. 1992. "Commercial Sex and HIV Risk: Male Partners of Female Sex Workers." Paper presented at the Eighth International Conference on AIDS, 19–24 July, Amsterdam.

de Bruyn, Maria. 1992. "Women and AIDS in Developing Countries." *Social Science and Medicine* 32, no. 3: 249–62.

de Caso, Laura Elena, et al. 1992. "Qualitative Analysis and Linguistic Methodology for the Design of Education Material for AIDS Prevention among Commerical Sex Workers." Paper presented at the Eighth International Conference on AIDS, 19–24 July, Amsterdam.

De Graaf, Ron, et al. 1992. "Heterosexual Prostitution Networks in the Netherlands and Britain." Paper presented at the Eighth International Conference on AIDS, 19–24 July, Amsterdam.

de Zalduondo, Barbara O. 1991. "Prostitution Viewed Cross-Culturally: Toward Recontextualizing Sex Work in AIDS Intervention Research." *Journal of Sex Research* 28, no. 2 (May): 223–48.

Dorfman, Lori E., Pamela A. Derish, and Judith B. Cohen. 1992. 'Hey Girlfriend: An Evaluation of AIDS Prevention among Women in the Sex Industry." *Health Education Quarterly* 19, no. 1 (Spring): 25–40.

Douglas, Mary. 1986. *How Institutions Think.* Syracuse, N.Y.: Syracuse University Press.

Ehrenreich, Barbara. 1983. *The Hearts of Men.* Garden City, N.Y.: Doubleday.

Ehrenreich, Barbara, and John Ehrenreich. 1971. *The American Health Empire: Report of Health PAC.* New York: Vintage.

Ehrenreich, Barbara, and Deirdre English. 1973. *Complaints and Disorders: The Sexual Politics of Sickness.* Old Westbury, N.Y.: Feminist Press.

Ehrenreich, Barbara, Karen Stollard, and Holly Sklar. 1983. *Poverty and the American Dream: Women and Children First.* Boston: South End Press.

Elifson, Kirk, Jacqueline Boles, and Lynda Doll. 1992. "HIV Seroprevalence and Risk Factors among Clients of Male and Female Prostitutes." Paper presented at the Eighth International Conference on AIDS, 19–24 July, Amsterdam.

Estebanez, Pilar, et al. 1992. "HIV Prevalence and Risk Factors in Spanish Prostitutes." Paper presented at the Eighth International Conference on AIDS, 19–24 July, Amsterdam.

Fleck, Ludwig. 1979. *The Genesis and Development of a Scientific Fact,* ed. Thaddeus J. Trenn and Robert K. Merton, trans. Frederick Bailey and Thaddeus J. Trenn, forward by Thomas S. Kuhn. Chicago: University of Chicago Press.

Fleming, Alan. 1988. "Prevention of Transmission of HIV by Blood Transfusion in Developing Countries." Paper presented at the Global Impact of AIDS Conference, 8–10 March, London.

Friedman, Samuel R., et al. 1992. "HIV Seroconversion among Street-Recruited Drug Injectors Who Have Sex with Women." Paper presented at the Eighth International Conference on AIDS, 19–24 July, Amsterdam.

Gallois, Cynthia, et al. 1990. "Preferred Strategies for Safe Sex: Relation to Past and Actual Behavior among Sexually Active Men and Women." Paper presented at the Sixth International Conference on AIDS, 20–24 June, San Francisco.

Gashau, Wadzani, T. L. Hall, and Norman Hearst. 1992. "Awareness Regarding AIDS and HIV Seroprevalence in Nigerian Long Distance Truck Drivers." Paper presented at the Eighth International Conference on AIDS, 19–24 July, Amsterdam.

Gilmore, Norbert, et al. 1992. "A Worldwide Survey of HIV/AIDS-Related Entry Restrictions." Paper presented at the Eighth International Conference on AIDS, 19–24 July, Amsterdam.

Haour-Knipe, Mary. 1992. "EC Concerted Action 'Assessment of the AIDS/HIV Prevention Strategies': Migrants and Travellers." Paper presented at the Eighth International Conference on AIDS, 19–24 July, Amsterdam.

Hassig, Susan, et al. 1989. "Contraceptive Utilization and Reproductive Desires in a Group of HIV-Positive Women in Kinshasa." Paper presented at the Fifth International Conference on AIDS, 4–9 June, Montreal.

Hawkes, S. J., et al. 1992. "A Study of the Prevalence of HIV Infection and Associated Risk Factors in International Travellers." Paper presented at the Eighth International Conference on AIDS, 19–24 July, Amsterdam.

Heller, Anne Conover. 1987. "Is There a Man in Your Man's Life?" *Mademoiselle*, July, 134–35, 153–54.

Hendricks, Aart. 1990. *AIDS and Mobility*. Copenhagen: WHO Regional Office.

Herold, Edward, et al. 1992. "Canadian Tourists and Sexual Relationships." Paper presented at the Eighth International Conference on AIDS, 19–24 July, Amsterdam.

Hughes, Veronica, et al. 1992. "Perceptions in the Use of Lubricants among Prostitutes." Paper presented at the Eighth International Conference on AIDS, 19–24 July, Amsterdam.

Hunter, Joyce, et al. 1992. "Sexual and Substance Abuse Acts That Place Lesbians at Risk for HIV." Paper presented at the Eighth International Conference on AIDS, 19–24 July, Amsterdam.

"In the Grip of the Scourge." 1987. *Time*, 16 February.

Johnston, Jill. 1973. *Lesbian Nation: The Feminist Solution*. New York: Simon and Schuster.

Juarez, I., et al. 1992. "Prevalence and Determinants of HIV and Other STDs in a Population of Female Commercial Sex Workers in Mexico City." Paper presented at the Eighth International Conference on AIDS, 19–24 July, Amsterdam.

Kane, Stephanie. 1989. "HIV, Heroin, and Heterosexual Relations." *Social Science and Medicine* 32, no. 9: 1037–50.

———. 1990. "AIDS, Addiction, and Condom Use: Sources of Sexual Risk for Heterosexual Women." *Journal of Sex Research* 27, no. 3 (August): 427–44.

Kaplan, Mark, et al. 1989. "Pregnancy Arising in HIV Infected Women While Being Repetitively Counseled about 'Safe Sex'." Paper presented at the Fifth International Conference on AIDS, 4–9 June, Montreal.

Kiereini, Eunice Muringo. 1990. "Women and Children in Africa: AIDS Impact." Keynote address at the Sixth International Conference on AIDS, 20–24 June, San Francisco.

Kramer, Jane. 1993. "Letter from Europe: Bad Blood." *The New Yorker*, 11 October, 74.

Kumaresan, Ganesan, et al. 1992. "Safer Sex for Truckers: Puzhal Tamilnadu." Paper presented at the Eighth International Conference on AIDS, 19–24 July, Amsterdam.

Latour, Bruno. 1988. *The Pastuerization of France.* Cambridge, Mass.: Harvard University Press.

Latour, Bruno, and Steve Woolgar. 1986. *Laboratory Life: The Construction of Scientific Facts.* Princeton: Princeton University Press.

Levine, Stephen B., and David P. Agle. 1987. *Intimacy, Sexuality, and Hemophilia.* New York: Hemophilia Foundation.

Lee, Chun-Jean. 1989. "Address." *Human Retroviruses and AIDS.* Proccedings of the symposium, 11–13 November, xii–xiii.

Lee, Ho-Chin, et al. 1989. "Update: AIDS and HIV-1 Infection in Taiwan, 1985–1988." *Human Retroviruses and AIDS.* Proceedings of the symposium, 11–13 November, 61–70.

Lyotard, Jean-François. 1988. *The Differend: Phrases in Dispute.* Trans. Georges Van Den Abbeele. Minneapolis: University of Minnesota Press.

Magana, J. Raul. 1991. "Sex, Drugs, and HIV: An Ethnographic Approach." *Social Science and Medicine* 33, no. 1: 5–9.

Mason, Patrick J., Roberta A. Olson, and Kathy L. Parish. 1988. "AIDS, Hemophilia, and Prevention Efforts within a Comprehensive Care Program." *American Psychologist* 43: 971–76.

Masters, William, Virginia Johnson, and Robert C. Kolodny. 1988. *Crisis: Heterosexual Behavior in the Age of AIDS.* New York: Grove.

McKeganey, Neil, and Marina Barnard. 1992. "Female Prostitution and HIV Infection in Glasgow." Paper presented at the Eighth International Conference on AIDS, 19–24 July, Amsterdam.

Moody, Dunbar T. 1988. "Migrancy and Male Sexuality in South African Gold Mines." *Journal of South African Studies* 14, no. 2 (January): 178–93.

Nejmi, Slimane. 1986. *Migration and Health.* Geneva: World Health Organization.

Nelson, Alvin, et al. 1990. "Characteristics Associated with a Low Return Rate for HIV Post Test Counseling among Clients in a Community-Based STD Clinic in Los Angeles County." Paper presented at the Sixth International Conference on AIDS, 20–24 June, San Francisco.

Nordheimer, Jon. 1987. "AIDS Specter for Women: The Bisexual Man." *New York Times*, April 3, 1, 10.

Norris, Barbara, et al. 1990. "Evaluation of Compliance Rate in a Clinic Serving Minority and Low Income Communities [Brooklyn, NY]." Paper presented at the Sixth International Conference on AIDS, 20–24 June, San Francisco.

Norwood, Christopher. 1985. "AIDS Is Not for Men Only." *Mademoiselle*, September, 198–99, 295–97.

Oliveira, Mariza Roedel, et al. 1992. "Truck Drivers: Evaluation of Attitudes and Knowledge in Relation to HIV/AIDS in Belo Horizonte, Brazil." Paper presented at the Eighth International Conference on AIDS, 19–24 July, Amsterdam.

Onorato, Ida M., et al. 1992. "High and Rising HIV Incidence in Female Sex Workers in Miami, Florida, despite Stable HIV Prevalence Rate over Time." Paper presented at the Eighth International Conference on AIDS, 19–24 July, Amsterdam.

Orubuloye, Olatunji I., 1992. "Sexual Behaviour, STDs, and HIV/AIDS Transmission: The Role of Long Distance Haulage Drivers and Itinerant Female Hawkers in Nigeria." Paper presented at the Eighth International Conference on AIDS, 19–24 July, Amsterdam.

O'Sullivan, Sue, and Pratibha Parmar. 1992. *Lesbians Talk (Safer Sex)*. London: Scarlett Press.

Painter, Thomas, et al. 1992. "Seasonal Migration and the Spread of AIDS in Mali and Niger." Paper presented at the Eighth International Conference on AIDS, 19–24 July, Amsterdam.

Panos Institute. 1989. *AIDS in the Third World*. Philadelphia: New Society Publishers.

Papaevangelou, G., et al. 1988. "Education in Preventing HIV Infection in Greek Registered Prostitutes." *Journal of Acquired Immune Deficiency Syndrome* 1, no. 4: 386–89.

Parker, Richard. 1999. *Beneath the Equator: Cultures of Desire, Male Homosexuality, and the Emerging Gay Communities of Brazil*. New York: Routledge.

Patton, Cindy. 1985. "Heterosexual AIDS Panic: A Queer Paradigm." *Gay Community News*, 9 February.

———. 1990. *Inventing AIDS*. New York: Routledge.

———. 1992. "Containing Safe Sex." In *Nationalisms/Sexualities*, ed. Andrew Parker, Doris Somer, Mary Russo, and Patricia Yaeger. New York/London: Routledge.

———. 1996. *Fatal Advice: How Safe-Sex Education Went Wrong*. Durham, N.C.: Duke University Press.

Patton, Cindy, and Janis Kelly. 1987. *Making It: A Woman's Guide to Sex in the Age of AIDS*. Ithaca, N.Y.: Firebrand Press.

Pheterson, Gail. 1990. "The Category 'Prostitute' in Scientific Inquiry." *Journal of Sex Research* 27, no. 3 (August): 397–407.

Pitt, David. 1990. "Potential Roles for Traditional Health Practitioners and Traditional Birth Attendents in National AIDS Control Programmes." Unpublished paper prepared for World Health Organization/Global Programme on AIDS consultation in Botswana.

Pizurki, Helena, et al. 1987. *Women as Providers of Health Care*. Geneva: World Health Organization.

Podhisita, Dhai, et al. 1992. "Social/Sexual Networks for HIV Transmission in Thailand." Paper presented at the Eighth International Conference on AIDS, 19–24 July, Amsterdam.

Portis, Suki. 1988. "Statement of the International Working Group on Women and AIDS." In *Cultural Activism, Cultural Analysis*, ed. Douglas Crimp. Cambridge: MIT Press.

Rabinowitz, Dorothy. 1990. "The Secret Sharer." *New York*. 26 February, 103–12.

Ratner, Michael. 1993. *Crack Pipe as Pimp*. Boston: Lexington Books.

Reardon, Juan, et al. 1992. "HIV-1 Infection among Female Injection Drug Users (IDU) in the San Francisco Bay Area, California." Paper presented at the Eighth International Conference on AIDS, 19–24 July, Amsterdam.

Richardson, Diane. 1988. *Women and AIDS*. New York: Methuen.

Richwald, Gary, et al. 1988. "Are Condom Instructions Readable? Results of a Readability Study." *Public Health Reports* 103, no. 4. (July–August): 355–59.

Rieder, Ines, and Patricia Ruppelt, eds. 1988. *AIDS: The Women*. Pittsburgh: Cleis Press.

Rifkin, Susan B. 1990. *Community Participation in Maternal and Child Health/Family Planning Programmes*. Geneva: World Health Organization.

Rosenberg, Charles E. 1962. *The Cholera Years*. Chicago: University of Chicago Press.

Russell, Michele A., et al. 1992. "The Perception of Risk for HIV Infection among Lesbians in New York City." Paper presented at the Eighth International Conference on AIDS, 19–24 July, Amsterdam.

Sabatier, Renée. 1988. *Blaming Others: Prejudice, Race, and Worldwide AIDS*. London: Panos Institute.

Sahraoui, D., et al. 1992. "AIDS Prevention Aiming at the North African Population Settled in Workers Centres." Paper presented at the Eighth International Conference on AIDS, 19–24 July, Amsterdam.

Salholz, Eloise, et al. 1990. "The Future of Gay America." *Newsweek*, 12 March, 20–26.

Sasse, Hartmnt, et al. 1992. "Potential Routes of HIV Transmission among Women Engaging in Female to Female Sexual Practices." Paper presented at the Eighth International Conference on AIDS, 19–24 July, Amsterdam.

Schneck, Mary, et al. 1989. "Reproductive History of HIV Ab+ Women Followed in a Prospective Study in Newark, New Jersey, USA." Paper presented at the Fifth International Conference on AIDS, 4–9 June, Montreal.

"Special Report on AIDS." 1985. *Newsweek*, 12 August.

Stall, Ron, et al. 1990. "Relapse from Safer Sex: The AIDS Behavioral Research Project." Paper presented at the Sixth International Conference on AIDS, 20–24 June, San Francisco.

Stephens, P. Clay. 1988. "U.S. Women and HIV Infection." *New England Journal of Public Policy* 4, no. 1: 381–402. Reprinted in *The AIDS Epidemic: Private Rights and the Public Interest*, ed. Padraig O'Malley (Boston: Beacon, 1988).

Sunderland, Ann, et al. 1989. "Influence of HIV Infection on Pregnancy Decisions." Paper presented at the Fifth International Conference on AIDS, 4–9 June, Montreal.

Taylor, Deane. 1990. "The Evolution of Dignity: Role of the Cook County Hospital Support Group for HIV Infected Women." Paper presented at the Sixth International Conference on AIDS, 20–24 June, San Francisco.

Treichler, Paula A. 1988. "AIDS, Homophobia, and Biomedical Discourse: An Epidemic of Signification." In *AIDS: Cultural Analysis/Cultural Activism*, ed. Douglas Crimp. Cambridge: MIT Press, 1988. First published in *Cultural Studies* 1, no. 3: 263–305.

Van Duifhuizen, Rinske, et al. 1992. "AIDS and Mobility: The Impact of International Mobility on the Spread of HIV/AIDS, Need and Possibilities for International Cooperation." Paper presented at the Eighth International Conference on AIDS, 19–24 July, Amsterdam.

Vernon, Diane. 1992. "A Prevention Program for Tribalized and Urban Bush Negroes." Paper presented at the Eighth International Conference on AIDS, 19–24 July, Amsterdam.

Vorakiphokatorn, Sairudee, and R. Cash. 1992. "Factors That Determine Condom Use among Traditionally High Users: Japanese Men and Commercial Sex Workers (CSW) in Bankok, Thailand." Paper presented at the Eighth International Conference on AIDS, 19–24 July, Amsterdam.

Wallace, J. I., et al. 1992. "Fellatio Is a Significant Risk Behavior for Acquiring AIDS among New York City Streetwalking Prostitutes." Paper presented at the Eighth International Conference on AIDS, 19–24 July, Amsterdam.

Ward, Helen, et al. 1992. "Commercial Sex and HIV Risk: A Six Year Study of Female Sex Workers." Paper presented at the Eighth International Conference on AIDS, 19–24 July, Amsterdam.

Wekker, Gloria. 1987. "Mati-ism and Black Lesbianism: Two Idealtypical Expressions of Female Homosexuality in Black Communities in the Diaspora." *Journal of Homosexuality* 24, nos. 3–4: 145–58.

Weniger, Bruce G., et al. 1992. "The HIV Epidemic in Thailand, India, and Neighboring Nations: A Fourth Epidemiologic Pattern Emerges in Asia." Paper presented at the Eighth International Conference on AIDS, 19–24 July, Amsterdam.

Whiteside, Alan. 1988. "Migrant Labor and AIDS in South Africa." Paper presented at the Global Impact of AIDS Conference, 8–10 March, London.

Wieringa, Saskia. 1989. "An Anthropological Critique of Constructionism: Berdaches and Butches." *Homosexuality, Which Homosexuality?* In Dennis Altman, Carole Vance, Martha Vicinus, Jeffrey Weeks, et al. Amsterdam: Shorer.

Wilke, Martin, and D. Kleiber. 1992. "Sexual Behavior of Gay German (Sex-)Tourists in Thailand." Paper presented at the Eighth International Conference on AIDS, 19–24 July, Amsterdam.

Williams, Glen. 1990. *From Fear to Hope.* Strategies for Hope Series, no. 1. London: ACTIONAID.

Wirawan, D. N., et al. 1992. "Sexual Behavior and Condom Use of Male Sex Workers and Their Male Tourist Clients in Bali, Indonesia." Paper presented at the Eighth International Conference on AIDS, 19–24 July, Amsterdam.

Wiznia, Andrew, et al. 1989. "Factors Influencing Maternal Decision-Making Regarding Pregnancy Outcome in HIV Infected Women." Paper presented at the Fifth International Conference on AIDS, 4–9 June, Montreal.

"Women and AIDS." 1987. *Time,* 27 April.

Women's AIDS Network. 1986. *Lesbians and AIDS: What's the Connection?* San Francisco: San Francisco AIDS Foundation.

World Health Organization (WHO). 1985. *Women, Health, and Development.* A Report by the Director-General. Geneva: World Health Organization.

———. 1987. *Evaluation of the Strategy for Health for All by the Year 2000.* Vols. 1–7. Geneva: World Health Organization.

———. 1988. *From Alma-Ata to the Year 2000: Reflections at the Midpoint.* Geneva: World Health Organization.

———. 1989a. *Broadcaster's Questions and Answers on AIDS.* Geneva: World Health Organization.

———. 1989b. *Report on the International Conference on the Implications of AIDS for Mothers and Children.* Geneva: World Health Organization.

———. 1989c. *The Reproductive Health of Adolescents.* Geneva: World Health Organization.

———. 1990. *The Work of WHO, 1988–1989*. Biennial report of the Director-General. Geneva: World Health Organization.

———. 1993. *World AIDS Update, Winter*. Geneva: World Health Organization.

Worth, Heather. 1998. "The Authenticity of Semen: AIDS, Sex, and Nostalgia, or Mourning the name of 'AIDS.'" Paper presented at the AIDS Impact Conference, Melbourne.

Index

Cindy Patton has been involved in AIDS community organizing, cultural analysis, and education since 1983. She has worked as a consultant to the World Health Organization and as a field ethnographer on an HIV study for the Centers for Disease Control. She has published numerous books on HIV and on sexuality, including *Fatal Advice, Inventing AIDS,* and *Queer Diasporas* (coedited with Benigno Sanchez Eppler).